Content

For my kids:
Nalini, Roshan, Savita, Ondine

Introduction

There are many excellent books on the anatomy and physiology of cells. This is the first book, however, devoted entirely to using mental imagery to improve the health of your cells, with emphasis on firsthand experience and practice. This book features the Franklin Method. What makes the Franklin Method unique is the specific effect of the power of thinking and dynamic physiological imagery on your physical state. Over the past 25 years, I have written many books on mental imagery, but here, for the first time, we will take it down a scale, to the cells of your body: the basic building blocks of your being.

The Franklin Method approach can be applied to any movement to improve it's function. My goal is to create happy minds and healthy bodies using ***Dynamic Neurocognitive Imagery (DNI)*** ™.

Dynamic Neurocognitive Imagery (DNI) ***™*** combines knowledge and research from a variety of fields including anatomy, kinesiology, biomechanics, and neuroscience. Using the DNI approach, we have developed tools and approaches for imagery use, which are being implemented nowadays in many universities, dance academies and sports organizations around the world.

The DNI research team is constantly working on investigating various aspects of the beneficial effects of DNI on human motor performance; this team is composed of specialists in the fields of imagery, biomechanics, and motor performance.

The correlation of health and imagery has been studied for years by the largest research centers worldwide, such as the National Institutes of Health in the United States. The power of imagery has shown successful application in sport, dance, and exercise (see Franklin, 2014 and Franklin, 2014). Today's athletes excel through their sophisticated use of mental imagery and related mental skills.

Founded by Eric Franklin in 1994, the Franklin Method makes use of movement, dynamic imagery, anatomical and physiological embodiment, and educational skills to create lasting positive change in your body and mind. The Franklin Method is taught all over the world, including the University of Vienna in Austria, the universities in Cologne and Karlsruhe in Germany, the Juilliard School, and New York University. The Franklin Method is recognized by health providers in Switzerland and is regularly presented at dance, Pilates, yoga, and physiotherapy conferences throughout the world.

CHAPTER 1

The Power of Imagery

One of the greatest discoveries of the 21st century is that the lives we live shape the brains we develop, referred to as the plasticity of the brain. The Franklin Method is at the forefront of practical neuroplasticity, showing you how to use your brain to improve your body's function. Starting with the knowledge that we have the power to change, the Franklin Method teaches you how to harness the transforming power of the mind to move your body with maximum efficiency and keep your body youthful and energized. A special focus of the Franklin Method is learning how it can be applied to improve all of your abilities.

"If you want to change your body, start by changing your mind." (Eric Franklin)

Research has shown that the most effective way to create changes in your brain is to change your thinking. Such mental interventions influence your immune system and organs in a positive way. These tools are free and always available to you, and have only beneficial side effects, so let's learn how to use them well.

Thinking, mental imagery, and physicality interact. *We become what we imagine*, and our imagination reflects our physical state. It is a two-way street. As your body represents the images and words present in your head, your mind will adapt to your posture, movement coordination, and tension level. A hurdler who is trained in mental imagery can visualize jumping the hurdles quickly and elegantly, making it to the finish line victoriously. A long-distance runner employs imagery to produce a sensation of "flow," the feeling of "running without trying." Thus, the running experience becomes a meditation, a prayer to the body's cells, so to speak. Science has repeatedly shown how imagery is a successful athlete's number-one mental skill (Feltz and Landers, 1983; Murphy, Nordin, and Cumming, 2008; Richardson, 1967b).

Negative imagery is powerful, too! While trained use of positive mental imagery goes hand-in-hand with achievement-oriented thoughts and actions, a body that is slouched and of low tone will accompany slouched and low-tone thoughts. Many people muse about their excess weight, sagging skin, weak muscles, wrinkles, or hair loss. They seem to be unaware of the fact that through such negative mental training, they are creating exactly what they don't want. This effect depends on the amount and strength of the negative thinking; it isn't about prohibiting negative thoughts dogmatically. If we only matter-of-factly become aware of our lack of abdominal tone and decide to do something about it, there will be no counterproductive effect. If, however, we decide to continuously obsess about our flabbiness but don't do anything about it, the negative imagery will assist in the body's adaptation to these thoughts, with the result of increased flabbiness. This mental display serves as a transmitting station to the cells.

Some people may consider negative thoughts to be motivating. For example, a fear of being unattractive can result in a person starting to go to the gym, albeit with apprehension and fear rather than enjoyment. Fear strongly encourages negative mental training, however. When one is terrified, one distinctly visualizes things one doesn't want to happen. The basis of effective mental training consists of a clear positive image, physical sensation, and emotional fortification. All of these are present during fear as well as rage, but in a very negative way. If one were to use the same elements to create positive images with positive emotions attached to them, the results would be very pleasing. Although visualizing the skin cells as clear, free, firm, and flexible may be a challenge at the outset, with time, you can learn how to use imagery with conviction and physical percipience. Everything takes practice; imagery is no different: Your skill will increase with the number of times you practice.

What Is Embodiment?

Imagery's role in your physical well-being occurs through your experience of embodiment. Embodiment is a physical insight that may be experienced as an improved sense of the enjoyment that accompanies a moving body. Referred to as a kinesthetic image, such an image is not just visual but is also felt in the body. It is a sensed knowing (a physical *aha!*) rather than an intellectual understanding. It is as if the body is communicating with you directly and telling you about its best function. A mental insight, rather than a physical one, may be a precursor to having an embodiment and may arouse the curiosity necessary to arrive at an embodiment, but it is not an embodiment. Embodiments can be likened to very clear images, often visual and kinesthetic. Once you experience the physical sensations evoked by the imagery, you realize that your previous knowledge about the benefits of the image was merely intellectual.

Types of Imagery

Imagery falls into a variety of types. Below are brief introductions to these types, to which we will refer throughout book.

Imagery can be spontaneous (arising from oneself) or programmed (obtained by an outside source). Spontaneous imagery originates from the person imaging in the sense that the person is the creator of the image, which may arise seemingly with no reason. Sometimes, spontaneous imagery arises from the use of another image. Often, a spontaneous image arises through the study of anatomy, literature, or the visual arts. Because spontaneous imagery is very personal, it is often highly effective. If a dance teacher has spontaneous imagery, he should be aware of this personal nature of the imagery before presenting it to his students.

Programmed imagery is imagery that is learned from an outside source such as a teacher, a book, or a recording. This general type of imagery is also used in teaching exercise and yoga.

Getting Stronger Without Moving

Mental simulation of movement (MSM) or mental rehearsal is commonly used in sports and exercise. When performing MSM, you are imagining doing a movement without actually physically moving. This affords the opportunity to rehearse and perfect a movement without the physical effort involved. MSM prepares your brain for performing the target movement, and mentally simulating a movement has an effect on your muscles, even though you are not volitionally moving at all. You can test this on yourself by imagining that you are bending and stretching your elbow. Even though you are not actively moving, you may nevertheless feel a slight activation of the muscles that are involved in elbow flexion and extension. The elbow that is mentally rehearsed will now feel more smooth and effortless in its action compared to the other side. MSM has even been shown to cause gains in strength, so one gets stronger without moving (Ranganathan et al., 2004)!

Biological Imagery

Most of the imagery in this book is biological, which can be subcategorized into anatomical, biomechanical, and physiological imagery.

When using anatomical imagery, you are imagining the structure and design of your body or movement. If you are visualizing your hip joint or imagining your lungs being flexible and free as you breathe, you are using anatomical imagery.

Biomechanical imagery involves precise imagery of the movement and forces occurring within your body. Even though it may take some practice to master biomechanical imagery, using your mind to imagine the physical mechanics of your movement will add smoothness and precision to your experience of moving.

Physiological imagery references the chemicals, hormones, and fluids of your body. If you imagine your blood swirling in the blood vessels or your electrolytes as balanced, you are using physiological imagery. This book provides an ample source of physiological imagery.

With biological imagery, the key is to focus on the process of anatomical change rather than on that which makes you unhappy or uncomfortable. If your shoulders are tense, for example, you can focus on the muscles lengthening and melting, rather than remaining stuck on the focus of what you do not want—in this case, tension. This may be a challenge in the beginning, but with time, you will become better at keeping your focus on what you want to create rather than on what you are not happy with. You can visualize all aspects of human anatomy: bones and joints, muscles and organs, fascia, the nervous system and the cells. Biological imagery can be useful if you understand that anatomical, biomechanical, and physiological imagery is not about becoming a walking anatomical lexicon but rather about improving your health.

Metaphorical Imagery

This book contains an abundance of metaphorical imagery. You are using a metaphor when you use an image or idea typically used to describe one object to describe another one. A metaphor is a kind of comparison. Metaphorical imagery is often easier to understand than biological imagery and can be used with all skill and age levels. The disadvantage of metaphorical imagery is that it is personal in nature; a metaphor that works for one person may be ineffective for another. It is therefore helpful to discover one's own favorite metaphors.

Metaphorical imagery has a tendency to morph or seamlessly change from one form to another. Allowing it to do so is part of your unique self-expression. You can combine metaphors with MSM. An example would be to imagine your arm moving like a feather floating in space.

Evolving Imagery, Seed Imagery

Imagery can change, or morph, between the metaphorical and biological versions quite seamlessly, with the aim of retaining the precision of the biological imagery and the quality of the metaphor. Morphing imagery works best with metaphors that resemble the anatomy they represent. The image changes from biological to metaphorical and back to retain the precision of the anatomical image and the quality of the metaphor.

Images can also evolve from each other. The first image in such a series is a seed image. In this case, you start with one image and notice how it evolves and changes as you move.

Key types of imagery are presented below in Table 1a, and Table 1b depicts the benefits available with different types of imagery.

Table 1a: Types of Imagery

Spontaneous Imagery	Imagery that is intuitive in nature arising from an inner source
Programmed Imagery	Imagery suggested from the outside
Biological Imagery	Imagery of the biological reality of the body in motion. Its three types, anatomical, biomechanical, and physiological, are described below.
Anatomical Imagery	Images the body structure as it is designed (the shape of the scapula) and/or how it moves (elastic responsiveness of the lungs' alveoli during breathing).
Biomechanical Imagery	Relates to the laws of motion and force in the body as contained in the basic laws of Newtonian physics.
Physiological Imagery	Relates to hormonal, chemical, and fluid functions of the body.
Metaphorical Imagery	Uses an image or idea that is typically used to designate one object to designate a different object. The image may bear little or no relation to human biology.
Mental Simulation with Metaphors (MSM)	Images an actual movement while adding a metaphor to create a desired quality. In this case, the metaphor, rather than the direct anatomy, performs the movement.
Morphing and Evolving Imagery	Images a seamless evolution from one metaphor to the next, or switches between the anatomical and metaphorical versions.
Seed Imagery	Uses an image to create other images, to foster creativity.
Sensory Imagery	Includes kinesthetic, tactile, visual, auditory, olfactory, and gustatory imagery.

Spontaneous Imagery	Personalized
Programmed Imagery	Provides a wide array of images to try
Biological Imagery	
Anatomical Imagery	Embodying function improves function
Biomechanical Imagery	Excellent choice to improve alignment in dance technique.
Physiological Imagery	Imagining a strong immune system or good blood circulation, for example, helps internal processes.
Metaphorical Imagery	Adaptable and personal. Within reach of those who lack the vocabulary for biological imagery. Freeing the imagination and invigorating the body, it can improve movement coordination, motor control, and quality of movement.
Mental Simulation with Metaphors (MSM)	Allows rehearsal of a movement without the physical effort involved, so good for practice when movement is constrained and good to practice without reinforcing old patterns.
Morphing and Evolving Imagery	Allows the mind to experience change, which in turn allows it to more easily imagine the body changing and adapting to new circumstances
Seed Imagery	Provides a starting point for the blossoming of multiple perspectives, implications, and applications of body-mind connection
Sensory Imagery	Promotes a sense of being in the moment, particularly when several senses are simultaneously involved in imaging.

Imagery in Space

Imagery can be located in a variety of spatial configurations: inside your body, outside your body, everywhere, or localized in a specific place. Use of imagery in space needs to be distinguished from the concept of imagery perspective. You are using an inner perspective when you are performing imagery from the vantage point of being inside your body, and you are imaging in the outer perspective when you are watching yourself from the outside as if on a screen or on a stage. The inner vantage point does lend itself more to kinesthetic, felt imagery than does the outer perspective. After a description of the four special orientations available by considering the inner versus outer and local versus global perspectives, a summary is provided in Table 2 below.

Inner Local

If you imagine your shoulder blades sliding on your back like a slippery bar of soap, you are using an inner local image. This image switches between the anatomical shoulder blade and the metaphorical bar of soap to catch the precision of the anatomical image and the movement quality of the metaphor.

If you imagine your hip joints, you are using an inner local anatomical image. If you imagine your spine bending from side to side like a shaft of wheat, you are using an inner local metaphor.

Inner Global

Inhale and imagine your whole body being filled by your breath. This is an inner global image. If you imagine snowflakes swirling around inside your body, you are practicing an inner global metaphor. If you imagine all the cells of your body, the image is inner global and anatomical.

Outer Local

If you imagine catching a ball, you are using an outer local image. The ball is in a certain place as it moves towards you.

Outer Global

An example of an outer global metaphor is imagining yourself floating in water and feeling the gentle waves nudging you from all sides.

Table 2: Examples of Imagery in Space (see Franklin, 2012)

	Inner	Outer
Local	See a soft feather floating between your shoulder blades, relaxing all the shoulder muscles. Imagine the center axis of your body. Imagine your hip joints.	Imagine a bird flying over your head. Imagine a tree on a hill. Imagine someone else in the room with you.
Global	Imagine your body to be filled with balloons moving you from the inside. Imagine the inner space of your body as intercon-nected. Imagine all your muscles to be flexible and strong.	Imagine yourself floating in water, feeling the gentle waves nudging you on all sides. Imagine yourself in the falling rain. Imagine yourself surrounded by beautiful flowers.

How This Book Can Be Used

All of my books are designed in a manner that makes it easy to visualize the body's processes and apply relevant imagery. By using illustrations to explain the material, I transform factual information into implementable imagery and embodiment exercises. With these exercises as a basis, you may also put together your own individual exercise sequences if that appeals to you more.

As you read over the pages of this book, you will notice its many illustrations. The aim of these illustrations is to inspire your imagination, not to constrict it. Feel free to embellish the imagery to your own liking. Often, you can benefit from the content of this book simply by gazing at the imagery and embodying it.

This book may be used in three different ways:

- **As a picture book:** Scroll through it, let the images have their effect on you, get inspired, and let yourself be moved and positively embodied.

- **As an exercise book:** Read through the exercises (they are highlighted) and try what appeals to you.

- **As a source for more knowledge about your body and for more comprehension of the connection between mind and body:** Read the introduction and explanatory paragraphs preceding the exercises.

CHAPTER 2

The Secret of Your Somatic Cells

The human body consists of five trillion cells, an inconceivable number. These cells are about 1,000 times smaller than the objects in your normal world, such as a lamp. Your cells produce everything essential to living out of the oxygen and food absorbed by the body: proteins, energy, hormones, and more. They serve as living recycling stations and mend your body after an injury. Any type of pain and every tension you experience is dependent upon the cell's condition. Cells are able to move and have their own skeletons. They are active and intelligent. They achieve connections, and they communicate amongst each other in a manner that makes any modern telecommunication seem primitive. This book explains how we can get in touch with our cells in a positive health-giving way. The goals are rejuvenation, health, power, confidence, vitality, and well-being. Your physical existence begins with the cell.

The instruments to create the changes we desire are always available to us: imagination and movement. Modern science tells us that thoughts influence the body through a cascade starting in the brain and moving through neuronal connections, cells, molecules, and, finally, genes. Over time, the heart's health matches the mood created by our recurring thoughts. The fitness of one's blood vessels adapts to one's level of stressful or non-stressful perception of one's world. Well-being is the immune system's barometer. Our physical, emotional, and mental behaviors create the environment in which our cells reside, and, by doing so, these same influences affect our genetic makeup. Our brain cells regenerate if we move our bodies amply and with joy. Even just 20 years ago these statements would have sounded rather esoteric, yet today, because of the emerging sciences of neuroplasticity and epigenetics, they are no longer taken so lightly. The field of inquiry into mind-body-mind influence has come of age.

A large part of the way in which we influence our cells takes place below our level of awareness—unconsciously and automatically. Even so, our intention and our efforts at understanding our bodies and our minds matter. We can decide to support our cells with the words we speak internally and externally, with imagery and empathy; doing so, we get in touch with the living building blocks of our bodies.

You are a unity of cells collaborating to create what you consider to be you. Is it worthwhile to become aware of your constituents? Satprem (1982) quotes the Mother in the book *The Mind of the Cells*: "Now I see. ... It would be like a unity, a unity made of innumerable—billions, you know—innumerable bright points. A *single* consciousness—made of innumerable bright points conscious of themselves. But it's not the sum of all the points! It's not that, not a sum; it's a unity. But an innumerable unity" (section 68.86).

Positions for Exercising

Many of the exercises in this book can be done while moving, others seated, and some reclined. Don't be surprised if you feel tension in a particular spot that doesn't seem to have anything to do with the area of focus. We often feel a reaction in the areas where we are the most tense at the time, even if the exercise is focusing on something else. As you continue practicing, this tension will melt away and leave you with a feeling of integrated well-being.

To practice Constructive Rest in the supine position, lie down with your knees angled at 90 degrees. Your feet are positioned solidly on the ground, and your legs are aligned parallel to each other (see my books *Inner Focus, Outer Strength* and *Dance Imagery for Technique and Performance*). Advantages of Constructive Rest include relief for your back and easier flow of blood to the heart.

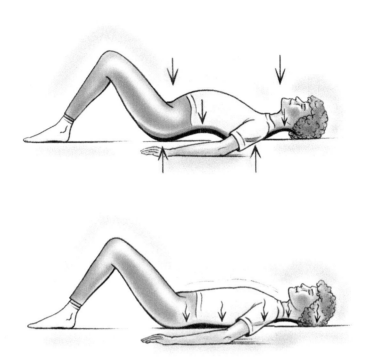

Cells in Comparison with Sand on the Beach

The human body consists of many different types of cells, all originating from a single fertilized egg. The cells in your body today have developed through a complex transformation called differentiation. This process is taking place all the time as new cells are born. In the marrow of certain bones of your body, one or two million new red and white blood cells are produced every second. The red blood cells, or erythrocytes, are responsible for transporting oxygen in the blood. The white blood cells, or leukocytes, are an important part of the immune system.

Before we take a closer look at the cells' composition and tasks, however, let's begin our journey to the inside of the body with our first cell imagery exercise.

Imagine your bone marrow in your sternum, vertebral bodies, and pelvic bones. Here, every second, more than one million new blood cells are born. Say to yourself, rhythmically, each second: "One million new cells, now another one million, a million, a million, a million." Think, "My body is infinitely creative; I am a cell millionaire, a cell billionaire! I am rich in healthy cells; I am getting richer in every moment. I live in abundance in every moment, automatically, without effort, simply rich in cells."

Illustrations 2 through 5 may help you imagine the large number of cells in your body.

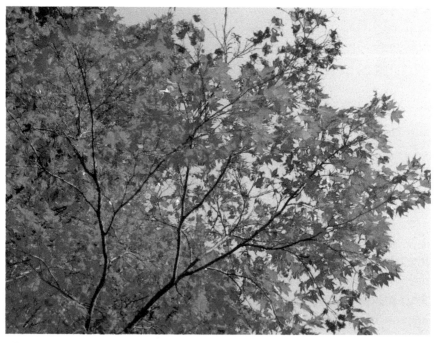

Illustration 2: Cells imagined as leaves fluttering in the wind

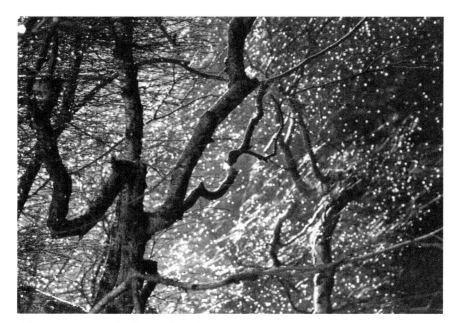

Illustration 3: Cells as dewdrops

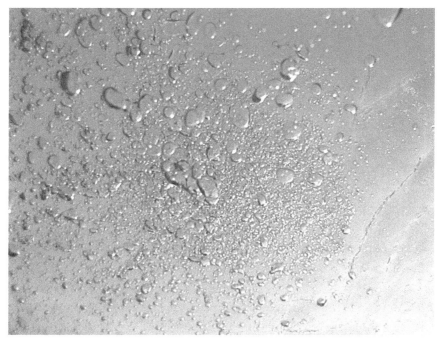

Illustration 4: Cells imagined as bubbles in water

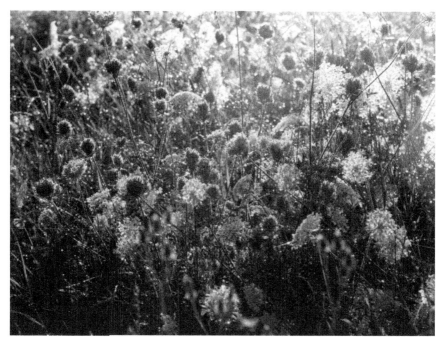

Illustration 5: Cells imagined as sparkles of light

Home Is Within Your Cells

Because we consist of an inconceivable number of cells, feeling at home in our cells ought to come to us naturally. The intention of the following visualization is to bring us closer to this idea.

I visualize one of my cells to be a comfortable apartment. The apartment contains beautiful carpets on the floor (or hardwood floors, depending on your taste), elegant furniture, paintings and pictures on the walls, and perhaps other especially charismatic pieces of art. I envision the apartment of my dreams precisely how I want it to be, with many nice things in it as well as having a pleasant atmosphere.

Now I invite someone into this apartment: a charismatic person whom I care about a lot. It can be a person I know or an invented fantasy person. I feel how the cell is filled by this person's positive energy. The person walks around in the cell and provides the cell with a sense of well-being. Everything the person touches within the cell begins to glow and becomes more radiant and beautiful. I now feel how all of my cells are being inhabited by this wonderful energy. There is simply no room for negativity in the cells. They are occupied by a juvenescent, mindful, beautiful, and healing being.

Infinite Layers

In nature there are eukaryotic cells, which include plant and animal cells, and prokaryotic cells, which comprise the two additional types: bacteria and archaea. Prokaryotic cells are unicellular organisms, usually bacteria, without nuclei or organelles. Prokaryotic cells typically live in large colonies. Plant and animal cells are not as different from each other as one may expect. Both plant and animal cells have a nucleus and organelles, for example. The cell wall of a plant cell is composed of cellulose, making it rather tough, whereas the cell wall of an animal cell is a very intelligent barrier that can allow or hinder the passage of a variety of substances.

Today, cells are basically synthesized in the same way they were billions of years ago. How the first cell or the first single-celled life-form evolved is heavily disputed. Contemporary theories consider whether cells originated in the earth's pre-biotic oceans, which formed a "primordial soup," or whether there was a spontaneous generation of cells by primordial mud.

Unfortunately, the evidence for the evolution of cells is missing. One can't track their origin. For example, in the evolution of mammals, cells suddenly appeared. Your own body cells are descendants of the first cells. From a cellular point of view, we are unthinkably old. The secret of the cells' origin rests hidden within them.

Every cell has a skin (cell membrane) and content made of fluids and solid substances (cytoplasm). Cells are composed mostly of fluids (70%), with the remainder composed of proteins, nucleic acids, ions, and other molecules. The inside of a cell is an area of bustling activity, filled with many enzymes for making and breaking the molecules needed for growth and energy production. The cell also contains DNA

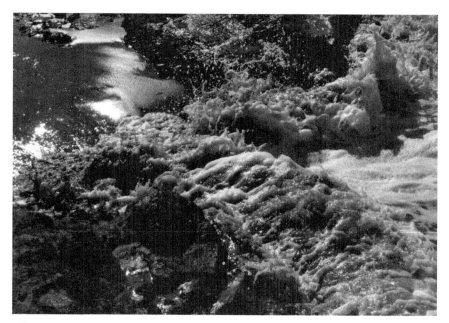

Illustration 6. Were the first cells created in the mud and pre-biotic bubbling of the oceans?

and ribosomes for building proteins based on the information contained in the genes. These processes we share with the animal kingdom. The difference between humans and animals is not so much in the genes, the neurotransmitters, or the way in which nerves conduct; we are all using the same machinery that was created eons ago. What is unique about humans is the way we activate this machinery—our ability, for example, to use mental imagery to create new possibilities for ourselves: possibilities that currently do not exist but that we would like to bring into reality.

The cell's membrane is double-layered and by no means firm. The membrane is a double-phospholipids layer that is semi-liquid like the "floating" surface of a bubble. Fluids, proteins, and molecules can make their way through this intelligent barrier. The area between the two layers of this membrane is called the periplasmic space.

Within the cell are smaller compartments containing specific molecular machinery. This was not always the case. The first bacteria-like cells (prokaryotic cells) came into existence approximately 2 billion years ago. About 1.5 billion years ago, a more modern cell appeared. In a bacterial cell, all the content is jumbled together, whereas in a modern eukaryotic cell, small separate compartments exist within which special functions are performed. These smaller compartments are called organelles. The organelles allow for a greater increase in efficiency in the cell. Individual tasks such as protein synthesis and energy production can be sequestered to the organelles, without their activity interfering with other processes. If you were to travel through the cell, you would encounter the nucleus, where the genetic information is stored; the endoplasmatic reticulum, a protein-production area; the Golgi apparatus, a sorting station; and energy-production facilities called the mitochondria.

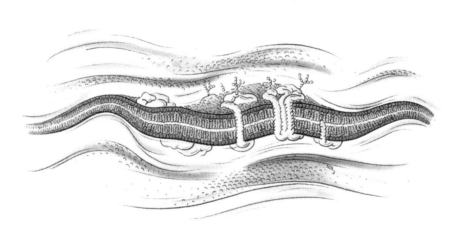

Illustration 7. Double-lipid cell membrane

The cell membrane is a distinct barrier through which only specific particles can pervade. It is an "intelligent" wall. The cell membrane is a place where intensive exchange takes place, and it is filled with channels, pumps, and sensors. In any given second, the cell is exchanging millions of bits of information with its immediate environment, with other cells, or with remote regions of the body. This information is brought to the cell as a messenger. For the cell to utilize the message, the cell requires a receptor, a docking place created specifically for the message.

One of the most famous and popular messengers is the endorphin, your inner opiate providing the message of well-being. Human beings are rather eager for the abundant flow of endorphins. During orgasm, for instance, the endorphin's rate of docking increases a hundredfold. Even without sex, endorphins can be stimulated, however, through relaxation and exercise. Endorphins are involved in the runner's high and in the general feeling of well-being after exercise. For example, dancers speak of luscious, pleasurable movement. Other messengers can also create motivation and a positive state of body and mind; these include serotonin, oxytocin, and dopamine.

Relaxing the Cell Membranes

Let's start by visualizing your skin, which is the largest membrane of the body. Let us use the metaphor of a big, water-filled balloon. Imagine the gentle movement of the water inside this balloon creating movement on the surface of the balloon. Imagine how the movement of the surface causes the water contained within to flow about. After a while, we cannot distinguish whether the water is moving the surface of the balloon or the surface is moving the water. We enjoy both sensations. Now let us imagine that there are smaller balloons within the big balloon, representing organs and tissues. Imagine the sensation of small balloons moving within the big balloon. Inside the small balloons are yet again even smaller balloons. Continue this image down to the very smallest balloons, which are the cells of the body. All balloons are permeable to water on this level, so we can travel along the waterways from one cell to the next.

Let's practice this image with the shoulders. First notice the current state of your shoulders. Maybe they feel a bit tight or rigid. Start by imagining your shoulders to be filled with water. (They actually are about 70% water). Gently move your shoulders and imagine water moving within in your shoulders, sloshing around as if the shoulders were water-filled balloons. Can you feel the liquidity within and around the cells in your shoulders? Can you feel fluid moving through the membranes of the cells of your shoulders? Imagine your shoulders to be permeable, an area of flow and transition. Drop any notion of compartmentalization and think of the shoulders being one fluid entity. Notice if your shoulders feel different now; maybe they have gained a sense of relaxation and ease.

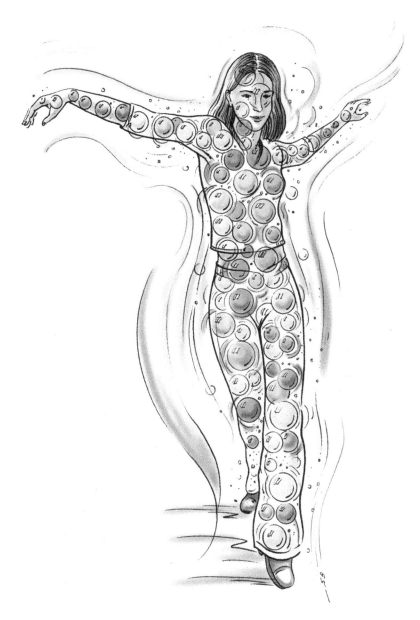

Illustration 8. Balloons inside the body

The Cell Membrane as Part of a Cloud

Imagine the cells of your body being soft, fluffy clouds. Move your arm or any part of your body, and imagine millions of small fluffy floating clouds. Move your spine, pelvis, and legs and imagine millions of fluffy floating clouds. Visualize the fluffy clouds providing lightness and ease to all areas of your body.

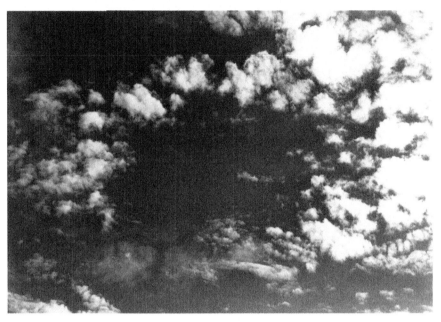

Illustration 9. A cell imagined to be a fluffy circular cloud

Visualize yourself floating through spaces in a fluffy cloud's membrane and immersing yourself in the fluffy cell. What does it feel like to be at the center of that cell? Imagine your awareness to be at the center of all your cells.

Your Cells Are Devoted

Imagine your cells busily working away, creating proteins, regenerating and protecting your body. Imagine every cell in your body devoted to your self-preservation. Imagine this attitude permanently existing within the cells. Imagine this devotion to a healthy body increasing within your cells. They don't question whether they should do their job. They always work with dedication. Their work is creative and fun. You can trust in the fact that the cells will do anything to keep you healthy. The willingness of your cells to give their all to keep your body running is so astonishing that it cannot be put into words.

Resting in the Cells

Imagine that centering your awareness within your cells is a comfortable and even cozy sensation. It feels like a deep inner meditation. Take notice if you can move while imagining this comfortable sensation of focus within your cells. When we are inside our cells, it feels as if we are everywhere in the body at once. It is not a matter of a fixed location; we are everywhere in the body at the same time because the whole body is made of cells. This is a true feeling of interconnectedness; it feels as if everything is relating to everything else. Can we move our bodies while being conscious of our bodies as a whole?

Cells with a Front Garden

As discussed earlier in this chapter, cytoplasm and a variety of organelles are inside our cells. We will continue this discussion later on, but first let's take a look at the cellular surroundings. Depending on the type of tissue, some cells are located next to each other, perhaps even touching, and others may be surrounded by a so-called matrix, a "garden" filled with the cells' "products." You can compare the two situations to a row of brownstone houses in a city street versus a country home with a garden.

Epithelial cells in your skin are located right next to each other, as are muscle cells. Connective-tissue cells have a garden that contains collagen, elastin, and glucosaminoglycans. The collagen provides tensile strength; the elastin provides elasticity, and the glucosaminoglycans maintain the hydration of the garden. Depending on the content of the surrounding matrix, the tissue may be, for example, cartilage, fascia, ligament, tendon, or bone. The garden matrix of the tendon cells is full of collagen, while the cartilage matrix contains lots of water. The collagen provides the tensile strength of the tissue, the water the resistance to compression.

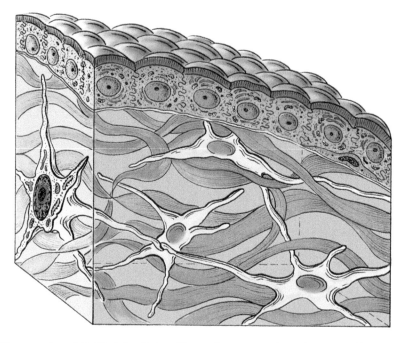

Illustration 10. Epithelial cells and connective tissue collagen

The brain contains neurons, and surrounding the neurons are astrocytes (star-like cells) as well as oligodendrocytes (cells with branches), which assist in the function of the neurons. These cells are grouped under the term neuroglia, or glial cells, from the Latin word *gliare*, meaning to glue. Interestingly, the term *neuron* is quite familiar to us, although astrocytes are more abundant in the brain. Originally, the astrocytes and oligodendrocytes were viewed as mere structural support and as secondary in importance to the neurons. Recent research has shown, however, that neuroglia are in fact very important for the function of the brain and that astrocytes seem to have a signaling capacity of their own, a function formerly thought to belong only to neurons.

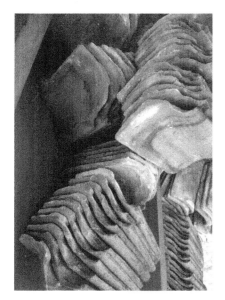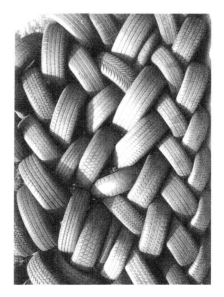

Illustration 11a and 11b). You can compare the arrangement of epithelial cells to an assembly of interlinked tires or roof tiles. Obviously, the quality of cells is quite different in these objects.

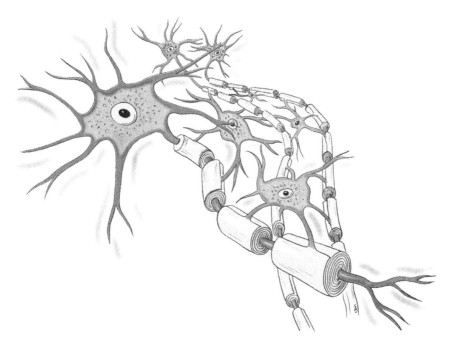

Illustration 12. Oligodendrocytes wrapping supportive myelin arms around neurons

Oligodendrocytes wrap an insulating sheath, called myelin, around the neuron, improving the function of the neuron. The shape of the oligodendrocytes gives them the appearance of being very busy protecting neurons, with many arms reaching out in all directions.

Inside a cell, you can find cytoplasm, the nucleus containing the genetic information, and other miniature organs of the cell, called organelles. Interestingly, the number of types of organelles in our cells roughly corresponds with the number of larger organs we carry in the body. The difference between the cell and the body as a whole is the great number of one type of organelles while we have only one liver and one stomach, for example. Depending on the cell type, the function of the organelle will vary, from cleaning duties, to protein synthesis, to librarian.

Enthusiastic Organelles

Imagine the organelles completing their work diligently and with much enthusiasm. If you think about the fact that your body contains about around 60 trillion cells, the number of organelles in your body is mind-boggling. Exact numbers do not exist, as no scientific endeavor has so far been able to accurately count the cells in body. (For more on organelles, see Chapter 2).

Liquid or Dry Environment?

Imagine your cells within their surroundings. How do you perceive this environment? Can you conjure an image of it? Is it hard and comparable to rock, dry like sand, or liquid as in the sea? Depending on whether we think of a bone cell, a muscle cell, or a cell within the watery intervertebral discs, imagining the cells' environment can truly be very different. In cartilage the there are few cells and a rich watery environment; in tendons the environment is many strong fibers. Epithelial cells in our skin hardly have an environment.

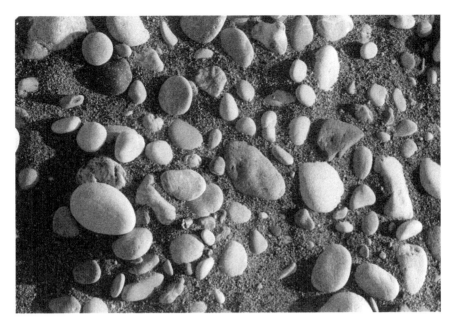

Illustration 13a. Cells as rocks in a dry environment

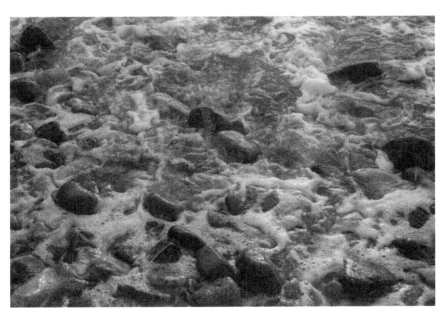

Illustration 13b. Cells as rocks in a liquid environment

Survival Through Companionship

Sometimes cells help each other out and protect one another from external impact. There are nursing cells in the thymus, and the aforementioned glial cells wrap themselves protectively around the nerve tracts, much like a mother who protectively hugs and nourishes her child.

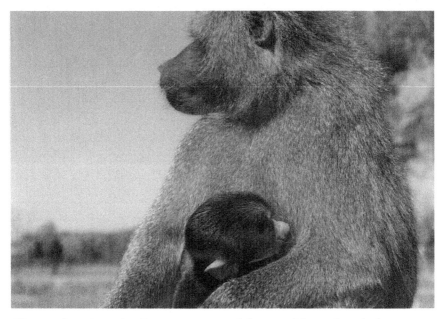

Illustration 14. Monkey mom nourishes and hugs her baby

Protozoa (single-celled organisms) were and are a successful type of life-form. They are especially abundant in water. Why is it that some cells have bonded to create a body? What are the advantages of living together? In a stable environment with abundant nourishment, there aren't any obvious benefits; however, as soon as food becomes scarce and the environment gets too cold, hot, or unstable, living together as a community has many advantages. The cells can supply each other with food; food can be stored; and layers of cells can protect important functions, reduce external impact, and provide warmth. Certain cells can also become experts on a single function. The advantages of working together as a community allowed more and complex cell bonds to develop and provide invariably better survival skills.

Empire penguins are a good example of mammals behaving like cells in a unit. To survive the arctic winter, the penguins group together to shelter each other from the biting winds and freezing temperatures. The outer penguins of the group serve as epithelial cells, so to speak, and the inner penguins are the heating unit, and by constantly cycling from center to periphery, all the penguins can stay warm. Their behavior also reminds us of the function of blood, which can both provide heat to distant areas of the body or serve to cool the body.

Cells Suspend Each Other or Support Each Other

Let your arms dangle loosely, and imagine how the cells are suspended from each other like a dense forest of pearl necklaces. If you lean on a table, however, the situation changes. When we prop ourselves up by our arms, we can imagine that the cells serve as miniature building blocks that provide support. Cells can also be visualized supporting each other laterally as they rest side by side, such as in the skin.

Many cells can, of course, do all the above functions to a certain degree; however, there are some major specialties, such as bone cells and the cells of muscles and connective tissue.

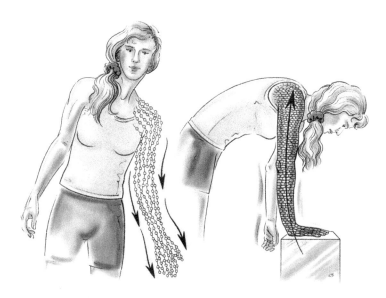

Illustration 15. Cells of the arm as dangling pearl necklaces or supportive building blocks

A Dive to the Cell Membranes

Our imaginary journey begins near the belly button. We imagine diving into our body through our skin. Initially the journey takes us through the different layers of the skin, then through layers of connective tissue, fascia, and a thin layer of fat. We may also encounter blood vessels, nerves and sensory organs in the skin. Next we dive through muscle. Muscles are surrounded and separated by connective tissue, so we may alternately encounter muscle tissue and connective tissue separations called septi and envelopes of fascia. As we go deeper we arrive at a layer called the peritoneum, which covers the organs. Below that we dive through the organ's capsule, deeply into the organ's tissue until we reach the cell membranes. After diving through the cell membrane we swim through the cytoplasm and discover the inner life of the cell.

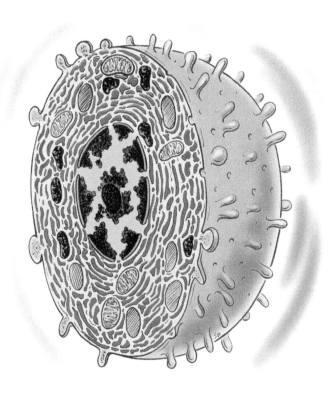

Illustration 16. Cross section of a cell with many membranes

Here we come across a multitude of membranes. These membranes surround the cell organelles.

The shapes of these membranes are very diverse. There are long membranes, and thick and thin membranes. There are oval and irregular structures with light or dark contents, with crystalline enclosures and bubble-like structures called vacuoles. We even discover a kind of skeletal structure of the cell and an active transport system.

Right in the center of the cell, we come across another membrane: the one that surrounds your nucleus. We dive through it and reach the DNA. This is your inner sanctuary, a library with assembly instructions that are at times copied to serve as blueprints to create proteins in the cell. What is created and copied depends to a great degree on your behavior, on how you move or do not move, and the kinds of emotions and mental activities you display.

We now slowly dive back up through the different layers, and finally we rest after this amazing journey through our own physical existence.

Taking Care of the Cell Membranes

What's taking place at the cellular level is pure dedication to your health. Without your being consciously involved, your cells aim to provide optimal function to all your tissues. The time has come to deliberately support this activity.

Imaginatively surround every cell with a touch of soft, protective energy. Imagine that the cells are being protected and supported by your consciousness. The cell membrane is being cleansed and cared for inside and out by a protective bright light.

Imagine that all processes in the cell membranes are of a positive and constructive nature. Joyful activity is taking place in the cell membrane, a joyful event in which only satisfied guests participate. Messengers such as the neurotransmitter endorphin bring the gift of well-being to the membrane while others contribute energy, beauty, and relaxation.

All products that leave the cell membrane aid your body, and everything that arrives in the cell provides cellular support. These exchanges at the cell membrane are governed by positivity. Each cell disperses its windfall to its environment near and far.

Finally, gently move any part of your body while maintaining some of the imagery described above.

Cells Breathe

The cell has a double membrane covering it, as do the nucleus and all the organelles. In order to discover all of these structures inside the cell, it is useful to first imagine cellular respiration. Cellular respiration is the process of exchange of oxygen and nutrients at the cell membrane. Oxygen that has found its way into the lungs hasn't reached its final destination. (This part of breathing is called ventilation.) Next, the oxygen needs to move from the alveoli of the lungs into the blood. Then the oxygen is carried through the blood by red blood cells to reach each and every cell in the body. Inside the cell, the mitochondria require oxygen to create the energy current of the body: adenosine triphosphate.

A fundamental goal for breathing is to breathe as deeply and thoroughly as possible. Your breathing should be adaptive and accompanied by a sense of ease and joy. Why not enjoy something you are doing about 20,000 times a day!

Thoughtful intentions or mental formulas may be very helpful in creating good breathing. In sports psychology, this is called *self-talk*; in yoga, it is referred to as a *mantra*.

Breathing with the Cellular Membranes

With sufficient practice, we may learn to imagine breathing with the different membranes of the cells. We start by imagining the breath of the inner membranes. Imagine the membranes as similar to the inner surface of the lungs.

Now imagine breathing into the space between the inner and outer membranes. Imagine this space to be wide and open. The perception of this space between the membranes may create a three-dimensional sensation. From this space, fluids, proteins, and other substances travel in all directions.

The breathing of the outer membrane is directed outward. Here, in the cells of the outer membrane, brisk exchanges of information are taking place. The cell membrane is a place of decision as to what to absorb and what to let go of. Imagine your breathing can take place in all of the outer membrane.

Notice if you have a tense spot in your body. Focus your cellular breathing in this area and see if you can dissolve the tension. Go deeper and deeper with your cellular breathing and simply exhale all the tension out of your cells.

Changing Behavior on the Cellular Level

Every human being has a specific behavioral pattern. Ideally, our behavior supports a healthier, happier life; however, we know this often isn't the case on a physical or psychological level. Emotions and mood states such as anxiety, anger, and depression have a deleterious effect on the cells of the body. What was dismissed by science until recently has been shown to be a key relationship: Emotional states and health are closely linked.

Stress is one of the unhealthiest emotional states to be in and fosters the production of cortisol, which weakens the cells. Cortisol is a hormone produced by the adrenal glands. It has the positive function of helping us out in truly dangerous and stressful situations. Sadly, as humans, we are able to continue feeling stress and to maintain elevated cortisol levels, even after any real danger is gone. We can cause stress simply through the images and thoughts crowding our minds. During prolonged stress, cortisol can reduce immune function, raise blood pressure, and increase craving for carbohydrates, resulting in weight gain.

Cognitive functions may be impaired, as well as bone regeneration, and eventually, our adrenals simply burn out.

One of the goals of performing imagery with our cells is to go in depth and discover the difference between a pattern and potential on the tissue level. We can break patterns and become open for something better and healthier. Through mental imagery, we can go directly to the adrenals, visualize the cortisol-producing cells, and imagine them relaxing and ultimately reducing cortisol production to healthy levels. Not surprisingly, dancing and laughing have been shown to reduce cortisol levels. Imagine your cells dancing and laughing right now, without even going to a dance class. In the best of all scenarios, you are actually dancing and laughing as you are imagining your cells doing the same (Berk, Tan, and Berk, 2008; Quiroga, Bongard, and Kreutz, 2009).

Candace Pert, the scientist who discovered endorphin receptors, says that we are capable of "thinking" on a cell-membrane level. Depending on which messengers the cell connects with, the cell perceives differently and differing reactions take place in the cell. When more endorphins are linked to the cell, we feel better. Given that we feel better, we also think differently. Everyone has had the experience that life moves along much more smoothly when we are in a good mood. The production of endorphins is enhanced by deep relaxation, and cellular breathing can lead to very deep relaxation (Kjellgren, Sundequist, Norlander, and Archer, 2001).

Studies point to the fact that higher levels of endorphins in the body imply better health and a stronger immune system. In other words, being happy and feeling good equals being healthy, which is hardly a surprise. The question becomes, then, one of identifying how we can produce a happier state in a regular and systematic manner (Panerai and Sacerdote, 1997).

Imagining Cellular Breathing

Cellular breathing, as unusual as it seems initially, is an anatomical image—in other words, biologically accurate and not metaphorical. To start with, it may be helpful to visualize respiration, the breathing in your lungs and the air moving through the thin membrane separating the capillaries carrying blood and the air in the lungs. You can then transpose this image to the cells, the difference being that you have two lungs and trillions of cells. You can also imagine the lungs' alveoli, miniature air sacks that can be likened to cells, breathing air in and out.

You may visualize one cell and imagine it breathing. The cells are actually taking in oxygen, then expelling CO_2 and free radicals. Even though this is true, it may be better to avoid the possible negative connotations of the latter two substances and to simply think breathing. Once you can imagine one cell breathing, start then imagining groups of cells breathing, then a whole limb or area of the body breathing, and then the entire body breathing.

When Cells Cough

Mental toxins for the cells are considered to be stress, fear, and panic, as well as negative, judgmental thoughts concerning oneself and others. Imagine the cells coughing up all these mental toxins and getting rid of them. When we think of our cells benevolently, we breathe with them; in turn, the cells will express their appreciation with healthy responses. Imagine that your cells appreciate your communicating with them. Imagine that your cells are happier when they aren't alone, simply toiling along without any recognition, but instead are receiving your support in the form of positive thoughts!

Ridding the Cells of Old Pain

Sometimes an old pattern of pain has gotten stuck in the cells. These cells may be tense because of a defensive mindset or an unhappy event in the past, though this mindset may not be relevant anymore and the problem long gone. Imagine telling your cells: "It's enough now; you can get out of this defensive state. You are allowed to breathe deeply again; relax and be happy." It may be that you immediately breathe more deeply after this inner assertion.

If we come across a spot in the body that doesn't breathe, we can go there in the mind's eye or feeling and ask those cells why they aren't breathing, what the problem is, and how we can help. Perhaps we see images such as dusty, dirty cells. Imagine these cells becoming clean and pure. Imagine them being washed out by pure and clean water.

Sponge and Jellyfish

Imagine yourself as a big sponge. This sponge is an accumulation of cells that functions as a unit and breathes as a whole body. Just like the cell, it absorbs water from everywhere and squeezes it out of its body again. For a couple of breaths, breathe through all your pores as if you were a sponge.

Now imagine you are a beautiful, toxin-free jellyfish, an animal whose relatively similar cells float easily and glide freely through its watery surroundings.

Two areas of your body that do float in liquid are the brain and spinal cord, so the area in which you think and perform imagery is actually floating. That should help your thoughts become lighter! You may remember a time when you let your body float in water, perhaps as a child in the bathtub or as an adult at some wonderful ocean beach. Two areas of your body are always on a beach vacation!

Breathing with the Whole Body

Lie down on the floor, using a mat or a carpet for comfort. Optionally, you may place a pillow beneath your knees and further pillows beneath your elbows. Ensure that the temperature is pleasant, there are no noises to distract you, and cell phones are turned off.

To begin, pay attention to your breathing. Notice movement caused by the breath. Most likely, you will feel this in the chest and stomach. Imagine the flexibility of the lungs, which expand elastically, and the relaxed movement of the ribcage.

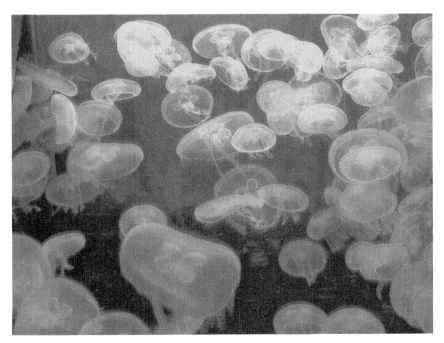

Illustration 17. Imagining floating jellyfish cells

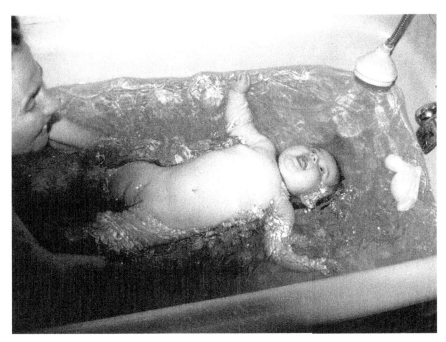

Illustration 18. A cell floats like a baby in the bathtub.

As you continue to breathe, you may notice other areas involved in breathing: the back, the shoulders, and the pelvic floor. Expand this sensation of breathing throughout the whole body, as if you were able to breathe with the whole upper body, torso and pelvis, legs, arms, feet, and hands. Soon, you experience your breathing all over the body as a subtle, soft expansion and contraction.

The diaphragm is a dome-shaped structure located in the lower part of the ribcage, and it moves downward as you inhale and upward as you exhale. Imagine the diaphragm floating; sense the diaphragm gently massaging the organs as it descends. On the inhalation, the stomach moves forward to make room for the organs. You may also feel the very bottom of the pelvis, the pelvic floor, expanding on the inhalation.

During exhalation, all of these actions reverse. The diaphragm moves up and you feel a pleasant stretching sensation in the fibers of the diaphragm. At the same time, the ribs float toward the center of the body as the lungs gently contract. The shoulders and facial muscles relax. The next inhalation follows effortlessly because of this complete exhalation.

Breathe for several minutes and observe these events without actively interfering. Imagine diving deeply into the body and into the middle of your cells. Imagine how respiration begins at the core of the cells. Imagine how it expands outward from this point through the cellular fluid, the cell membranes, and the body. Respiration is like a pleasant wave that envelopes the body with a smooth sense of well-being. Exhale, and the cells relax with a sense of contraction, yet without any collapse or loss of form.

Cellular Respiration with a Golden Light

In the supine position (lying on your back on the floor or a yoga mat), pay attention to your cellular respiration. Your breathing may create a sense of your body relaxing and melting like ice cream in the sun. Feel this sense of melting beginning in the head and slowly sinking though the body, relaxing all tissues.

Visualize a red-golden color flowing from the head into the body; this vibrant color fills every cell in the body. The cells absorb this color, and all of the cell's organelles and membranes turn red-golden. All cells are now surrounded by a red-golden glow, which is visible all the way to your skin. Inhale, and realize how this color improves your respiration and how inhalation intensifies the color. Don't exert yourself in seeing this color, but approve of it and admit it into your cells. Bathe in the pleasant sensation of the red-golden color. This color serves as a protection for your cells, which get strengthened as if by an elixir of life that gives eternal health. Nothing can harm your cells; they are now immune to any dysfunction.

Having this sense of safety in the tissue, breathe for a while and observe the colors in the body. Possibly, other colors will appear. Don't prevent this. Instead, become a calm observer. Perhaps you see your cell membranes glow in many different colors. Purple can show up in the front, but there are also pink and blue membranes. This gives the cells a colorful and peppy look.

After about ten minutes, start moving again and emerge from your healing breathing experience.

With a Partner: Cell Respiration in Motion

In this exercise, we work in pairs. The purpose is to feel the cellular respiration in movement.

The first person touches the partner's upper back and shoulders. Tap or rub the area to increase the cellular respiration into the tissue. After that, place your hands on your partner's shoulders, while your partner focuses the breath into the shoulders. Remain in this hand-to-shoulder respiration for a while, then the partner changes position. Choose another spot on the body to touch, and start the process over again. In every area, it's useful to imagine that the respiratory rhythm equals the cellular breathing rhythm.

Next, your partner initiates movement in the area where he or she perceived the cells breathing. In other words, the cellular breathing triggers the movement. Afterward, your partner begins moving continuously as you keep touching different body parts that trigger movement via cellular respiration.

After about 15 minutes of this exercise, the partner's body that was practiced on may feel transformed, and a deeper awareness of the cells and the breath may emerge. Switch partners, and repeat the exercise.

Flowing Cells

It wouldn't be too bold to claim that humans consist of liquid and membranes. The membranes are the body's inner borders. Water making up a variety of fluids is one of the most important means of transport and communication. Most membranes, such as the cell membrane, are permeable to fluids, whereas others, such as skin, are less so.

As we have already learned, the state of the body affects mental consciousness, and vice versa. A flowing feeling in our bodies imparts a mental sense of flow. Tension in the body tends to create a more rigid mental stance. Membranes allow us to experience both flowing and permeability, and sometimes more solidity as in a barrier. The later may be useful in situations where you feel the need to protect yourself from a harsh environment, both on an emotional and physical level.

When our thoughts stagnate, when we are lacking in inspiration, the membranes are likely to be tense. The sense of liquidity and softness is absent.

Hand Breathing with a Partner

Stand opposite your partner and pay attention to your partner's breathing. Touch the palm of one of your hands to the palm of one of your partner's hands. Imagine the hands as being two cells that are in contact with each other. Your skins are the cell membranes. The two cell membranes communicate with each other, send each other messages. The cells are filled with fluid, which supports communication. You send your messages with the help of this liquid through the membranes to the other cell. Allow for movement to occur. React to the movement and the breathing of your partner's cells. Breathe from your skin into your partner's skin. Be aware of your partner's cellular breathing; active communication is taking place. After about five minutes, break the contact. Let your arms and hands rest, and observe how your breathing and posture have changed. Partners can then switch roles.

CHAPTER 3

The Inner Life of Your Somatic Cells

What our bodies need, we take in through food, yet the proteins of our body are produced within the organelles. The cell organelles are basically miniature factories; they are the basis of all vital processes. The inner respiration, the metabolism, the production of proteins and enzymes, all of these take place within the organelles. The biggest organelle is the nucleus. Additionally, there are organelles with more exotic names: mitochondria, lysosomes, ribosomes, peroxisomes, the Golgi apparatus, and the endoplasmic reticulum (see, for example, Illustration 21). Vast numbers of organelles are present in our bodies. The imagery exercises in this chapter will help with incorporating the organelles into your health and fitness consciousness.

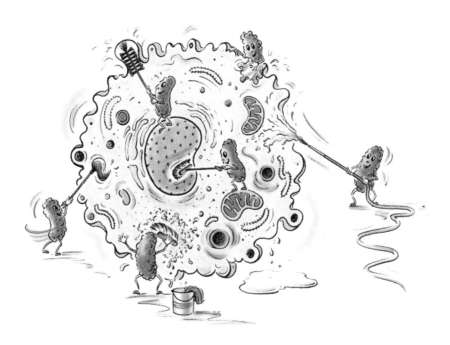

Illustration 19. Imagine your cells being scrubbed clean.

The Cell as a Solar System

Imagine the cell as a small solar system. Imagine it as an independent system with a central sun, the nucleus, and the planets (the organelles) all revolving around the sun. The sun and the planets are a harmonious team. All of the partners in this game are in continuous communication and exchange.

The Mitochondria

The mitochondria are the cell's energy-producing factories. Their output is adenosine triphosphate (ATP), the chemical energy source of the body. Where more energy is needed, a larger number of mitochondria are present. A liver cell has about 1,000 mitochondria, whereas an egg cell may have up to 20,000.

The mitochondria have double membranes. The inner membrane is heavily folded, making the surface area much larger. We can imagine this to look much like a row of densely folded curtains lined up in layers next to each other. This is where the actual ATP synthesis takes place. Mitochondria are the keystone between the digestive and respiratory apparatus. Oxygen and nutrients (glucose) come together here to produce energy. Water, ATP, free radicals, and carbon dioxide are all produced by the mitochondria. ATP is the body's most important medium of energy storage. Without ATP, not a single muscle movement would be possible.

Some diseases accompany malfunctioning processes of metabolism in the mitochondria. For instance, there is a disease that physically appears like an advancing palsy, in which excessive iron accumulates in the mitochondria. It acts like a poisoning of the mitochondria, which then fail to enable muscle movement.

Aging is associated with the mitochondria. Free radicals are a byproduct of energy production. An excess of these can lead to cell death and various diseases. What free radicals do, very simply explained, is steal atoms out of other tissues. This is much like removing stones from a brick building, making it unstable and in danger of collapsing. This is why foods rich in antioxidants are a healthy choice, because they aid in the prevention of these occurrences.

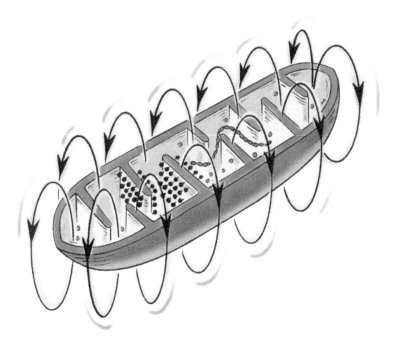

Illustration 20. Cross section of a mitochondrion

Cellular Springs

By imagining water being produced in our cells, we may help our bodies relax and feel more fluid in general. Place a hand on your shoulder, with your thumb touching your neck. Your hand is now placed on a muscle called the trapezius. You can visualize water being produced underneath your hand, a true biological image. Imagine the breathing of the cells. Imagine a gliding or sliding sensation between the infinitely many membranes of the cell organelles. The liquid between them provides softness and relaxation.

How can the shoulders, neck, or any part of the body be tense when millions of fresh springs provide a constant rejuvenating bath? Imagine how water cheerfully gushes from one cell to the next and millions of small bubbling ponds wash away all tension.

Fluidity in Your Shoulders

Let us now move the shoulder and imagine that we are moving the water within our shoulders. We are about 70% water, so why should our shoulders be exempt from feeling watery?

We hold up one arm without losing the liquid sensation. We lift the shoulder and let it drop very slowly, and feel the weight and flow of the water in the shoulder. Repeat the lifting and dropping several times.

Now repeat the action with the other arm. Hold up the arm with a liquid sensation, and lift the shoulder and let it drop very slowly. Feel the weight and flow of the water in the shoulder. Repeat the lifting and dropping several times.

We move our wrists in a circular fashion while slowly dropping our arms back down to our sides. When our arms are down, we enjoy the feeling of relaxed shoulders and take this wonderful sensation with us into our everyday lives.

The Mitochondria's Origin

The structure of the mitochondria is surprisingly similar to that of a bacterium. This is the basis for a theory, of how it came to be that we have mitochondria in our cells. Perhaps a very long time ago, a bigger cell engulfed a bacterium, and the bacterium remained in the cell and eventually took over the task of being the power plant of the cell. The mitochondria (originally a bacterium) now had the advantage of always having access to food, and no intricate chase for nutrition was necessary.

Mitochondria have their own genetic makeup, enabling them to split and duplicate. The only other organelles that function similarly are the peroxisomes. An interesting fact to note: The mitochondria are matrilineal, meaning the lineage of the mitochondria is thus traced to the mother, not the father. According to modern science, we are able to trace our mitochondria all the way back to a primordial mother in Africa.

Mitochondria are also trainable. As we age, the ability of the mitochondria to process oxygen and nourishment and to produce energy is reduced. This situation can be improved, however, through exercise. Active people have more mitochondria, and their mitochondria are fitter.

You may imagine the mitochondrion as an energized skipping Ping-Pong ball and imagine a low humming sound, a deep energy at the cell core.

Breathing with the Mitochondria

The body's deepest breathing takes place in the mitochondria. Imagining the mitochondria's respiration creates a sensation of global energy, elasticity, and relaxation.

In a relaxed standing position, stretch your arms upward and lower them down again very slowly. Inhale as you lift, and exhale as you lower your arms. Find a pace that feels comfortable for you. Throughout the movement, focus on the millions of respiratory entities in your cells. Imagine how breathing takes place in the mitochondria. In an everlasting cycle, the mitochondria absorb oxygen and give off energy. Feel how this energy flows through the tissue and nourishes it.

After several minutes, rest your arms and enjoy a relaxed sense of energy running throughout your body. Aim to maintain this sensation in your everyday life.

The Right Number of Free Radicals

Free radicals are one of the mitochondria's metabolic products. The mitochondria are responsible for the energy supply in the body, producing water, carbon dioxide, and free radicals. An excess of free radicals may lead to an accelerated tissue reduction.

In a comfortable supine position, take time to explore your body's inner consciousness. Ask yourself: "Are there areas that feel especially pleasant? Are there areas that feel tense? Where do I breathe deeply? Where am I most aware of my breathing, and where am I not aware of my breathing?"

Clear your mind of all thoughts. If thoughts are swirling through your head, simply let them flow out like a stream of water or imagine them turning to dust and getting carried away by a pleasant wind. Imagine that there is room only for constructive and nourishing thoughts.

Become aware of the rest of your body with its trillions of cells. Visualize the cell membranes, and imagine them becoming brighter. They emanate a glow similar to the illumination of a lampshade when the light is switched on. The membrane feels light and elastic.

In your mind's eye, continue floating through the cell and arrive at the energy-production site, the power plant, the mitochondrion. A pleasant warmth is emitted by this organelle, a feeling as if you were approaching a fireplace, with much anticipation, on a cold winter day.

A golden glow shines out of the mitochondrion. Inside the mitochondrion, oxygen and nutrients are being converted into energy. Feel how there is always plenty of oxygen available for your mitochondria and how your nourishment is converted thoroughly. Feel how there is plenty of energy available for your muscles and for all of your body's other structures. The free radicals are produced only to the extent necessary to support your body's recycling process. The mitochondria's ideal balance is established.

Remain in this comforting sensation for a while, and then dive out of the cell and back to observing your outer breath. Has it changed as well?

Take enough time to stand up slowly by rolling onto your side and resting for a moment before you get up.

Endurance, Thanks to the Mitochondria

We have a greater number of mitochondria in places such as the heart, where more energy is required. When an individual exercises, the inner membranes expand and the space between the outer and inner membrane becomes wider. This enables faster metabolism.

For individuals who run, swim, or participate in other activities that stimulate the cardiovascular system for a prolonged period of time, the following visualization may be helpful.

Visualize the space between the outer and inner membrane of the mitochondrion noticeably enlarging. The sensation triggered by this can be compared to the fluffing up of a pillow: If it was compressed and flat before, it now is now enlarged and stretched out. The mitochondria increase their capacity. You now suddenly feel like your endurance has increased.

I would like to reveal a personal experience I had using a similar visualization as described above. One day while swimming, I practiced visualizing the mitochondria. As I dipped my head underwater, I realized that I could hold my breath significantly longer, as long as I maintained my focus. Whales and dolphins, both able to stay underwater for prolonged periods of time, are possibly adept at this skill. They can control their mitochondria and thus produce less CO_2, or they may even have very large mitochondria.

The Endoplasmic Reticulum

The endoplasmic reticulum consists of a highly visible number of labyrinth-like corridors and passages. If we look at a glandular cell, we will see that it is usually packed with endoplasmic reticula (see Illustration 16), whose job is to produce hormones. If we visualize our endoplasmic reticulum, what we will see are membranes packed within membranes, which are yet again packed into more membranes.

There are two types of endoplasmic reticula: rough (RER) and smooth (ER), with both types consisting of cell membranes and a space between them. Sometimes this space is narrower, and, at other times, the space is wider and contains tubes, channels, and bubble-like vesicles. The endoplasmic reticulum fluently merges into the membrane of the nucleus. If you have been fortunate enough to visit there, imagine the channels of Venice. In contrast to Venice, the channels of the ER aren't consistent, and they can change their shape, creating discs, tubes, new channels, and bulges, as if Venice morphed and changed its layout every day. This would make it rather difficult for tourists—or anyone, in fact—to find their way around.

We can see that on the cellular level, human beings are superbly flexible and exist in a non-gravity environment, a floating world, where everything zips around and bounces into everything else to create reactions and new substances. No matter how tight you may feel in an area of your body, your cells remain flexible, pliable, and ever changing. If you can transfer that concept, feeling, and image to your body in general, you will start feeling very flexible and full of potential. You are very creative at all times on the cellular level.

You may argue that this is all a fantasy, yet you would then be denying your biology, because you *are* your cells. You are made of cells, and this is what is happening inside you! Can you feel your cells? We can turn this statement around and say cells are actually what we feel and that it is their activity, neuronal or other, that causes the sensations of the body.

The RER's surface is studded with little black dot-like structures called ribosomes, which give the RER a polka-dotted appearance. The ribosomes' products are dispensed into the RER. Imagine a conveyor belt with many little pastries on it, and here they wait for further transport along the pipelines of the RER. This isolation is important. In the case of an enzyme, it may cause damage or a premature reaction in the open cytoplasm of the cell. A few of the products made in the RER are destined for the lysosomes and peroxisomes. The others are bound for export.

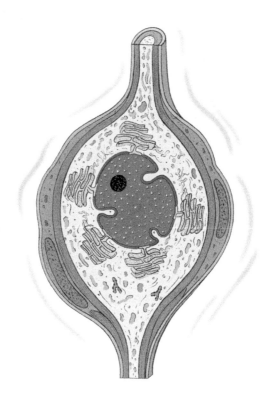

The RER also functions as an elastic, moldable conveyor belt for proteins. Plasmacytes are cells that belong to the immune system and contain a lot of RER. They are significant producers of proteins, specifically antibodies. There are a lot of smooth endoplasmic reticula in the plasmacytes, pipe-like constructions without ribosomes on the surface. Astonishingly, your cells are capable of producing one half million different proteins. At the cellular level, human beings are rapid and efficient protein factories.

Floating Towels

When I was a kid, sometimes the bath towel would somehow end up in the bathtub with me. If you have seen a towel floating in water, you know what I saw: a folded, floating and moving mass of softness. Here is the metaphorical image—visual, kinesthetic, and tactile—that we can use to develop our sense of the endoplasmic reticula: Floating layers, a complex landscape in the water, consisting of myriad folded membranes. Imagine the membranes as multiple towels floating in the water. If the water moves, the towels are being moved as well. If the towel moves, the water is stimulated as well.

The Membrane's Connectivity

We imagine that all of the body's membranes are connected to each other, from the endoplasmic reticulum's most inner membrane and the nucleus all the way to our skin. The membrane's connectivity enables the outer layers to lead to the inner layers, and vice versa. In this sense, all membranes are attached to the nucleus, which is quite an astonishing concept. We enjoy the holistic feeling of all areas of our body being connected through the membranes.

The Ribosomes

The ribosomes are perhaps the smallest factories ever, producing many vital proteins. One could argue that the body's existential interface, the keystone between our "blueprint" and physical existence, is located in the ribosome. The ribosome receives the blueprint to build proteins from the nucleus, which contains the genetic material in the form of mRNA messenger-ribonucleic acid. This blueprint then serves to build our proteins. The ribosome is where we come into existence, an exciting place to focus on!

Not all ribosomes sit on the RER. So-called free ribosomes, or polyribosomes, are distributed in the cytoplasm. Sometimes they are also connected by mRNA strands and float around in the cell like garlands. Free ribosomes, among other things, are responsible for the production of hemoglobin, which enables the red blood cells to absorb oxygen.

The mRNA contains all information used by the ribosome to produce proteins. The mRNA is the concept, the data from which we develop. The ribosome and the RER make up the factory that transcribes this concept. Thus, the ribosome is the doorway between the plan and our physical existence. Before the RER activity, our bodily structure exists solely as a blueprint. You may think that these functions cannot be influenced; however, we now know that this is not true. As mentioned previously, the body exhibits plasticity, changeability dependent on our behaviors—mental, emotional, and physical. If we change our behavior and the result is an increase in cells in certain areas of the brain and a remapping of neurons, the ribosomes have certainly been involved.

Energy for Your Ribosomes

It is important to first relax our bodies in order to best visualize the cells. We can do this through focusing our attention on sensations arising from our bodies, such as our breathing. We can also do this through movement. Move your shoulders in a circular path; first move them up, then to the back, then down and forward again. Breathe consciously as you do this. Stay focused on your movement, the breath, or both. After a minute or two, switch the direction of the circular motion.

Once you have performed these actions, you will notice that your shoulders are more relaxed and so is your mind.

Now imagine diving down through the different layers of the body all the way to a cell membrane. Sink deeper into the cell's interior and start recognizing the structures we have discussed previously. You can imagine the structures as being many different colors. You can visualize the ribosomes on the endoplasmic reticula, distributed like small points on winding membranes. Now imagine the blueprint information floating into the ribosome. Imagine that the information is used to produce beautiful and healthy tissues. Keep focusing on healthy production: the path from blueprint, to assembly, and to a magnificently created you. Imagine that this process is being influenced in the most positive way possible. Take responsibility for producing the very best you. Your tissues are constantly being replaced; imagine that the replacements are even better and more refined.

Smooth Skin, Thanks to the Loving Ribosomes

We now focus on different body parts: the ribosomes in the skin cells producing perfect skin proteins for smooth, beautiful skin, and the ribosomes in the joints producing perfect synovial fluid for flexibility and elasticity.

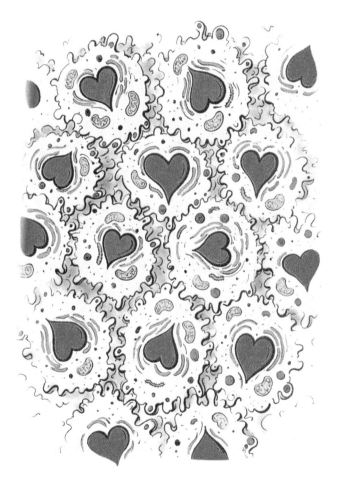

Illustration 22. "Love cells"

We visualize that the ribosomes, regardless of their locations in the body, produce with great joy and love. Proteins that are saturated with love are stronger and more resilient. It is well known that people who live in environments with other caring people tend to live longer, so now we can bring this sensation of a caring environment directly to the cells and ribosomes. We imaginatively write the word "love" onto the ribosomes and RER. This feeling spreads throughout the whole cell. The cells are in love with their task. We then feel deeply satisfied within our cells and bodies.

The Golgi Apparatus

The Golgi apparatus is named after Camillo Golgi (1843–1926), an Italian neurohistologist who discovered these organelles inside the neurocytes. The Golgi apparatus is basically the mail-order house of the cell, where wrapping, sorting, and product inspection take place. Most products need to be slightly amended and so take the time to ripen before they are sent away in small spherules, the transport vesicles. Inside the vesicles, the chemical ripening process can continue. Much like the process of making good cheese or good wine, the ripening of the proteins takes time.

The Golgi apparatus looks like multiple layers of inflated canvases stacked on each other. Each Golgi apparatus has a convex side and a concave side. The layers of the Golgi apparatus resemble double-walled buildings that aren't connected to each other but are aligned in terms of their shape. The Golgi apparatus's convex side is the absorption and growth side, while the concave area is the ripening and emission side. The edges are somewhat wider. Here we come across small transport vesicles. At any given time, an inconceivable number of transport vesicles are launched. We can visualize the vesicles separating from the Golgi apparatus's concave edge; like soap bubbles, they float off to their destination.

The imagery of transport bubbles floating freely can be useful as an inspiration for movement; however, it isn't entirely accurate. Within the cell, there are proper railways consisting of microtubules, which are attached from the center all the way to the cell's periphery. On these rails are little protein locomotives that are able to transport the vesicles. One type of locomotive, called dynein, is responsible for the transportation from the periphery to the cell's center at a kind of central station near the Golgi apparatus. Other locomotives, called kinesins, are responsible for the transportation to the periphery. The movement of these locomotives looks a lot like a caterpillar moving on a branch.

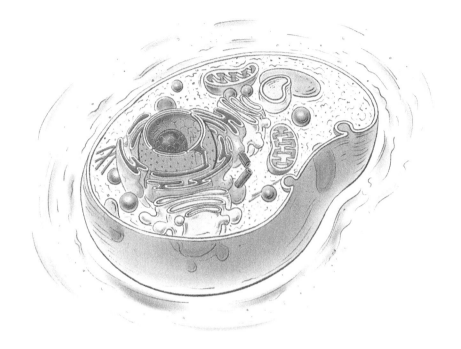

The endoplasmic reticulum delivers proteins to the Golgi apparatus, where the proteins are restructured. This conversion, among other things, consists of linkups of proteins with carbohydrates, as if individual pieces of fabric were to be sewn together into a dress. These linkups are used, among other things, as proteins or fat components (lipids) in the construction of the cell membrane.

The transport vesicles can also fuse with the membrane and get rid of their content outside the cell. Several vesicles may create a lysosome, which constitutes the cell's digestive and recycling system.

Vesicles

The best way to begin this visualization is to observe soap bubbles. Watch a bubble grow, separate, and float off. This is a rather precise, though much bigger, model of the action of the vesicles. Imagine now

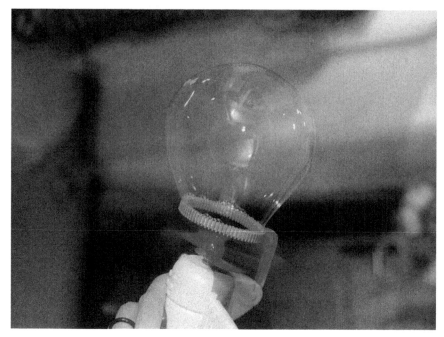

Illustration 24a. A vesicle compared to a soap bubble

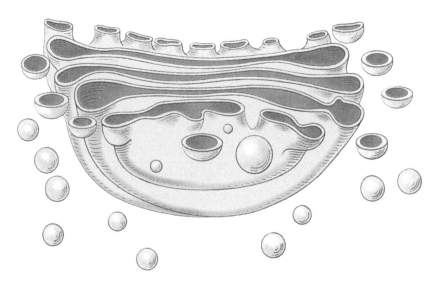

24b. Golgi apparatus and transport vesicles

that this occurs millions of times a second within your body and that, because of this activity, the constituents of your body are being distributed both inside and outside the cells. This image of millions of weightless bubbles floating around gives your entire body a sense of lightness and gives you a sense of floating *inside* your body. The vesicles are floating because the environment they are in, in practical terms, is weightless.

The bubbles can also travel through the cell membranes to reach neighboring cells. They are literally scooped up on one side of the membrane and ejected on the other side.

The Lysosomes

Lysosomes became known as separate cell organelles in 1955, and since then scientists have gained more and more understanding of their significance. The lysosome is a body enclosed by membranes and has an extremely acidic environment. Acidic enzymes are produced in the ribosome and then transported via the endoplasmic reticulum to the Golgi apparatus. Here, they are packaged into membrane bags and become lysosomes.

Lysosomes have different shapes; some are round and others oval. There are big ones with brighter contents and others with crystalline inclusions. They form the intracellular digestive system. They break down overage cell organelles, which are gathered up in vacuoles. The cell produces these vacuole trash bags to dispose of things that aren't needed anymore, and these vacuole trash bags are then digested by the lysosomes.

The lysosomes are very actively involved in the development of the organs in the embryo. For the development of organs tissue need to be created but also certain cells need to be dissolved. Here is an example: The embryo has webbing on its hands just like a frog, and this tissue helps the development of individual fingers. Scavenger cells that contain numerous lysosomes eventually digest away the excessive tissue.

The lysosome is the recycling factory and, in some aspects, acts as both the digestive apparatus and the kidney of the cell. The lysosome breaks down used cell parts into their constituents and passes them on to the cytoplasm's internal recycling system. The body's scavenger cells have a significantly high number of lysosomes to break down absorbed microorganisms. In the liver, the spleen, and the bone marrow, many of these cells are present. These scavenger cells are responsible for the decomposition of worn-out blood components, toxins, bacteria, and many other substances. The scavenger cells within the liver, the Kupffer cells, have a purifying function thanks to the lysosomes they contain.

In the lung are lysosomes in the alveolar macrophages, specialized "vacuum cleaner" cells that clear the lungs. The lungs are constantly exposed to dust and toxins entering as we breathe, so these macrophages are essential for the housekeeping of our lungs. Many lysosomes are also found in the adrenal glands, in the bone marrow, and in the spleen—everywhere in the body where a great deal of breakdown and digestion takes place.

When something is absorbed from the outside into the scavenger cells (phagocytosis) with the aim of being digested, it is initially packed into a membrane called a phagosome. This phagosome floats around in the cell until the lysosome has time to eliminate it, as if trash bags were floating around and the flying disposal units catch up with them one at a time. After everything has been broken down by the enzymes, residual bodies can develop; these are also called aging pigments. If several of them are present, sometimes a change in color, pigmentation, develops in the cell.

Disruptions in the lysosome lead to accumulations of waste products, just as if garbage collectors were striking. Several different storage disorders can cause such disruptions. Certain drugs can also prevent the lysosome's breakdown functions.

Lysosomes are closely related to the lymph system. The lymph circulation consists of lymph nodes and channels, which eliminate and dispose of bacteria, viruses, and cell fragments. The lymph is your inner cleansing system, and approximately 10% of the fluid returning to the heart returns through the lymph channels. When blood flows back to the heart through the veins, destined for cleansing, it is directed to the lymph channels. As in a water-cleansing facility, the fluid must be purified before it can return to regular circulation. The lymph system also functions to transport fats that have been absorbed from the digestive tract, giving it a milky appearance.

Cellular Inflammation Protection

The lysosomes eliminate all sorts of undesired matter from the cells by simply dissolving it. Their inner environment is corrosive, and they have a protective layer, called glycocalyx, inside the cell membrane. Lysosomes are part of inflammatory processes because a significant number of materials that are to be broken down develop during inflammation. I once experienced knee pain because of an inflamed knee bursa (a type of fat pad that facilitates the gliding of the tendon). When I imagined the lysosomes toning down their cleansing frenzy, my knee felt better instantly. A possible explanation is that an exaggerated reaction had occurred; the lysosomes had overly activated their corrosive contents.

The skeptic within me argued that this was a placebo effect or that my general positive outlook had created the healing! This specific visualization did do the trick for me, however, so why should I allow a skeptical mind to talk me out of something that helped me? Thinking that because you do not believe something is possible, you are not allowed to have the experience defeats the whole purpose of mental imagery.

Lysosomes rid us of everything we do not need. Imagine that everything the cell doesn't need any longer is absorbed and removed by the lysosomes. We can feel how our cells are being purified and cleansed. The cells feel lighter, the whole body is in equilibrium, and breathing is freer because oxygen doesn't need to be channeled through debris. The cells gleam with bright purity.

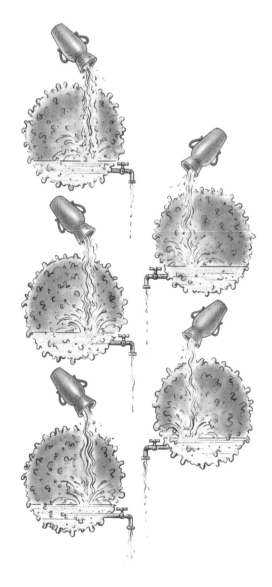

Building and Purifying the Cells

We will now focus on the areas within our body where there are things we no longer need, where things are being dissolved or where debris is being separated into its parts so it can be reused for new substances. These areas are the lysosomes, our miniature kidneys. The lysosomes attract cell fragments and parts that otherwise would disrupt the body's functioning. Like a first-class vacuum cleaner, the lysosomes absorb and remove all "cell dust," and as this happens, the health of our cells increases. What remains is a clean cell.

Imagine that the cell membranes absorb everything that is good for them and reject everything that is bad for them. The cells open up to love, peace, calm, well-being, energy, satisfaction, and relaxation. These emotions are poured into the cells like a refreshing elixir. All negative emotions such as hatred, jealousy, envy, anger, and avarice stay outside. These negative emotions are absorbed by scavenger cells and recycled so they can become food for positive emotions.

Feel how the cell membranes are permeable to positive vibrations; they widen themselves to receive these positive emotions. With every inhalation, absorb positive emotions, and with every exhalation, rid yourself of negative emotions. Visualize that every cell possesses an outlet through which it can excrete refuse. The cell eliminates all harmful matter while simultaneously replenishing itself with nutritious foods and emotions.

The Peroxisomes

The peroxisomes are not present in all cells. They vary in shape and are found in high numbers in the liver and kidneys, where they aid in breaking down fatty acids and uric acids. The breaking down of uric acid is important for the health of our tissue and especially our joints, to avoid a condition called gout. Peroxisomes are also key for the health of the brain and nervous system, as they manufacture plasmalogens, the most common phospholipid in the myelin sheaths surrounding the neurons. The peroxisomes were possibly the cell's first energy-delivery system, before this task was taken over by the mitochondria.

Dissolving Stiffness

Move all the joints in your right arm, in the shoulder and in the elbow, and imagine the peroxisomes actively supporting your ease and comfort in doing so. More and more, the feeling in your joints and tissues becomes elastic and unobstructed. If you feel any stiffness, imagine how this sensation is simply digested by the organelles, specifically the peroxisomes. The stiffness is literally dissolved from within.

Begin moving more and more of your joints, including the spine and your left arm. Feel how everything that may disrupt your movement is being dissolved and washed out of your system. You feel increasingly flexible, soft, and light. Imagine how the peroxisomes and the lysosomes are always working to improve your flexibility, making your body comfortable and supple for life. Using this mental imagery is like doing inner yoga asanas, stretches and gyrations of the cells, although we are not overtly stretching but are creating flexibility by embodying the inherent flexibility in the cellular matrix.

Healthy Myelin

Imagine that the peroxisomes are busily creating plasmalogens for a healthy nervous system. Visualize the nerves being wrapped in many layers of healthy sheaths, increasing the nerves' conduction rate, nutrition, and safety. Imagine you're the cells of your brain and your entire peripheral nervous system, magnetically attracting the perfect amounts of constituents for the protective myelin. Imagine your nerve conduction to be smooth and relaxed.

The Vacuoles

These transport vesicles have been mentioned several times already. They can be in transit through the cell, in a process called transcytosis, without directly getting in touch with it. In endocytosis, the vacuoles are being received and taken in by the cells. This occurs after extensive testing in the cell membrane. The cells can also dispense vacuoles, which is called exocytosis. These are the cell's gifts to the rest of the body. Glandular cells produce many vacuoles, whose contents of hormones are released into the space between the cells.

The Vacuole as a Travel Companion

Imagine yourself sitting inside a gigantic vacuole. This vacuole is your companion in your journey through the cell. Your task is to visit every organelle and to bring each of them encouragement, praising them for their good work. The goal is to create a feeling of movement and permeability through your whole body. All tension vanishes because tissues can be cleared and brought into communication with each other through the vacuoles.

Now notice how movement is taking place on the membrane, and notice how the vacuoles travel through. Imagine floating with the current and penetrating the cell membranes; gently float out and then back in again. Experience the cell's interior as a peaceful lake; as soon as you leave the cell, things become more active and there is more movement and directionality in the fluids. The currents become stronger; the feeling penetrates everything. All is liquid, flowing, with a sense of infinite penetration. Let yourself be carried by the vacuoles through the entire body and the cell membranes.

Notice how this imagery is affecting your sense of your body. How do you perceive your surroundings once you feel all this flow in your body? Has there been a change in the quality of your thinking?

The Cellular Skeleton

The cell has a dynamic and flexible skeleton, which is called the cytoskeleton. This skeleton can adjust itself quickly to any type of situation, and it can do it almost as quickly as someone putting together the Eiffel tower in Paris within a minute! This skeleton consists of the microtubule; the microfilaments, or actin filaments; and intermediate filaments. The highly variable structure is essential to the cell's shape and locomotion, as well as for the transportation of organelles and vesicles. If one were to compare a cell's composition and function with those of bones and muscles, the microtubule would be the bones, the actin filaments would be the muscles, and the intermediate filaments would represent the cell's connective tissue.

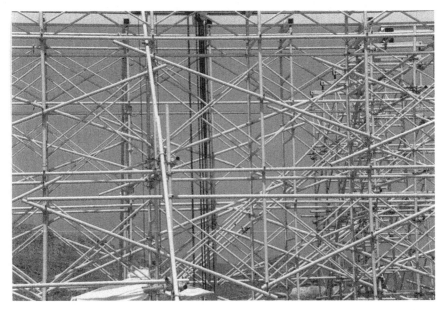

Illustration 26a. The cytoskeleton can be compared to a scaffold.

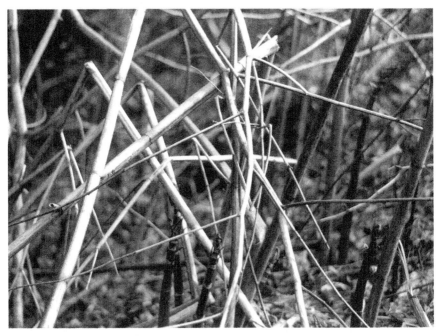

Illustration 26b. Microtubules crisscross the cell, similar to how these twigs cross each other.

The microtubules are basically the cell's steel pipes. They consist of individual parts called the tubulins, which are assembled similarly to the construction of a building. The finished microtubules are arranged in the cell either separately or in a bundle. They can also be taken apart very quickly, and the individual parts can be used repeatedly. We can imagine the microtubule much like poles in a tent: The cell membrane is the tent wall and is stretched out over the microtubule, the tent poles. If the microtubules are destroyed, the cell dies; in our metaphor, the tent has collapsed.

The Microtubules

Microtubules are the railway for the transportation of vesicular bubbles from the endoplasmic reticulum to the Golgi apparatus and all over the cell. The proteins dynein and kinesin serve as locomotives for this transportation. Imagine a caterpillar with a backpack moving across a branch: The branch is the microtubule, the caterpillar is the kinesin or dynein, and the backpack is the bubble.

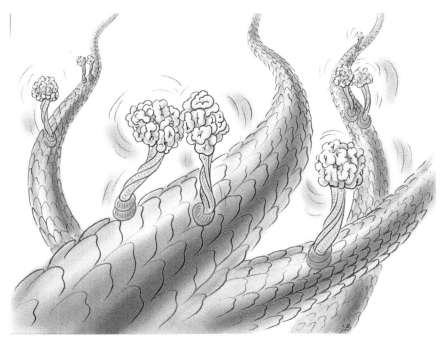

Illustration 27. Dynein walking on microtubule

Microtubules are also used as miniature "oars" in the cells, forming cilia, small hairy projections that the cell can wave back and forth. The cilia are often called flicker hairs and can be found in the lungs and the fallopian tubes. The cilia sway and bend rhythmically in a coordinated manner, looking somewhat like a cornfield being blown by the wind. In the fallopian tubes, the cilia move the fertilized egg toward the uterus. In the lungs, they remove soot, dust, and other unwelcome particles, moving those particles upward so they can be swallowed and digested. Smoke and air pollution cripple the cilia. The good news is that if someone decides to quit smoking, the cilia are capable of recovering fully.

A longer type of cilia is called flagellum and also consists of a microtubule. The sperm's tail projection is such a long flagellum, and the sperm uses it for propulsion.

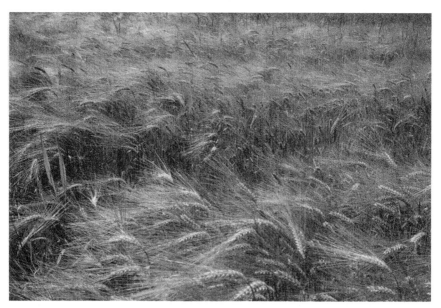

Illustration 28. Flagella move like wheat in the wind

The Centrioles

Every cell contains cylindrical centrioles. These are located near the Golgi apparatus at the organizational center, the microtubule's central station, so to speak. They consist of nine triple units of microtubules, each containing three microtubules. In most cases, centrioles come in pairs, with the longitudinal axis of one facing the other vertically, much like rods in a scaffold. The centrioles are essential to cell division. In preparation for this process, they duplicate, and they assist in organizing the genetic substance at the cell's poles.

The Microfilaments

Microfilaments can be compared with fine yet very strong spider webs. They occur as single threads or as netlike structures. Microfilaments consist of a roundish protein called actin, which reaches significant lengths particularly in muscle cells. In the muscles, the microfilaments, or actin filaments, work together with myosin to achieve muscle contraction. Actin and myosin are located in muscles, both in heart and in striated and smooth muscle. Striated muscle is what we typically consider a muscle, such as the biceps and gluteus, whereas smooth muscle is found primarily in the digestive system.

The Intermediate Filaments

In terms of size, intermediate filaments are midway between microtubules and microfilaments. They are responsible for stability, have great tensile strength, and can get very long. The nucleus is wrapped fishnet-like by intermediate filaments, which can spread from there all the way to the cell membranes.

With the help of these components, the cell forms a complex, stable, and variable structure in its interior called the trabecular micro-grid. This grid resembles the constructions of architect Buckminster Fuller, who named the underlying principle tensegrity. In a tensegrity, or floating compression, system, isolated components of compression, such as a beam, are located inside a net of continuous compression, possibly wires or elastic bands. This arrangement has the advantage of needing fewer and lighter parts than a conventional structure. It is nevertheless very sturdy and resilient because any kind of pressure is being received and distributed equally over the whole system, instead of being supported by individual parts. The skeleton is anchored to the extracellular matrix. To visualize this, let's revisit the tent metaphor. Think of the anchoring pegs and how they cannot just float in space. They are anchored, in the case of a tent, to the ground, and in the cell, they are anchored to the extracellular matrix, which we previously called the garden surrounding connective tissue (Ingber, 1998).

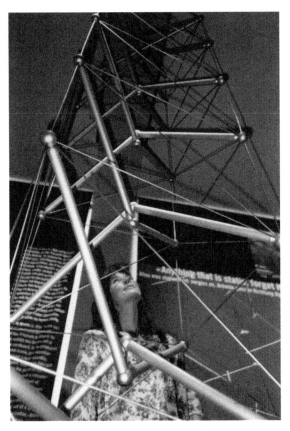

Illustration 29. Tensegrity tree

We also come across the tensegrity principle in the body's macro structure, as exemplified by the pelvis and spine and their ligaments and muscles. The cellular trabecular micro-grid surpasses even Buckminster Fuller's building in terms of its flexibility. It can expand, contract, and adapt itself to the cell's movements, almost like a house that could move along by growing a leg that simply pops out of a wall and connects itself to the ground or a surrounding object, and then that object drags the house along with it.

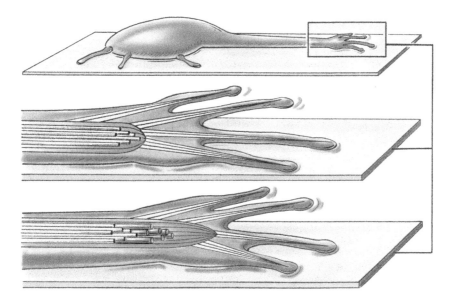

Illustration 30. A cell moving with the help of legs containing cytoskeletal components

No building can match its shape to the prevailing weather, though this would be useful. A building cannot diminish in size or expand to expose more surface area to the sunlight and heat itself. Many cells can do this and much more. In one instance, a cell may be flat, and then it may easily form into a round ball. If a cell lacks fluid, for example, the trabecular micro-grid contracts to ensure the cell's integrity. The grid can adapt its tonicity and serve as a diverse suspension device for ribosomes as well as other cell proteins. Thus, the body's fundamental tension integrity indeed is based in the cell.

Initially, cells in an embryo are undifferentiated; in other words, they have not yet defined their jobs and positions in the future body. When these cells of the embryo travel to their new destinations, they form legs, which are called pseudopodia. Within these legs, a skeleton is formed temporarily. With the help of these pseudopodia, the cells walk along fibronectin roads to their destination within the developing body.

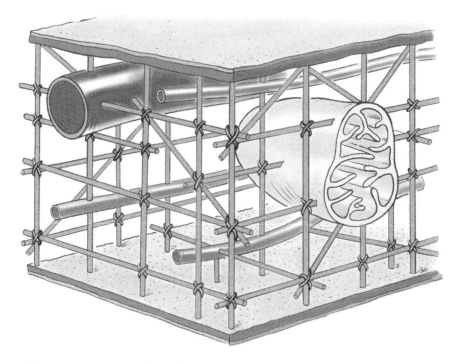

Illustration 31. Trabecular micro-grid as a suspension device for the cell's organelles

The cytoskeleton isn't merely a static skeleton but is also dynamically malleable and thus simultaneously serves as the cell's muscular system. Even more surprisingly, changes in the cell's configuration can alter gene expression; in other words, these genes are turned on to create proteins (Ingber, 1997).

Nothing but Flexibility

Perform any movement that comes to your mind—shrug your shoulders, lift an arm, or flex and extend your spine. Perform this movement again and focus on the cytoskeleton's perception of reality. This is an anatomical image, as cells do stretch and bend, flatten and widen in response to your movement. Every tissue needs adaptability, and in addition, the stimulation of the connective tissue induces the production of proteins. As you move, imagine your cells bending, stretching, folding, and widening. A sensation of suppleness is present all over your body. Initially, this may be a mental stretch, as we are so conditioned to think that our muscles power the movement in joints. The cells must change somewhat as you move; it's a fact of your biology.

If we feel tension anywhere in the body, we become conscious of the fact that this tension can be changed into flexibility in a matter of seconds. Imagine the cytoskeleton expanding, relaxing, and becoming more flexible or making room for more fluid. Perceive tension as a momentary imbalance in the cytoskeleton rather than a permanent condition in the muscle. Believe that all tension can change into sense of flow and ease.

Lifting Weights with Cytoskeletal Imagery

From a cellular point of view, your body consists of a trabecular micro-grid triangle constituting the tensegrity of your body. This is a most stable structure, able to easily endure a lot of weight. It does not bear the weight like a wall by resisting, however, but rather through the stretch of the tensile elements. This is a good idea, as it is more efficient to endure a lot of pressure through tensile rather than compressive means.

Because imagery is about orienting our focus toward something that is valuable and useful, let's focus in the cytoskeleton as we lift a weight. Instead of simply focusing on a set of muscles, focus cellularly to engage the force of all the cells involved in lifting. On a deep level, if you imagine tensegrity, lifting an object is not a push but a stretch. At first this may seem unusual, but it is based on anatomy, and with time, we may embody this concept.

Practice the following: First lift a weight by focusing on activating muscles. If you don't have a dumbbell, simply use a heavy book. Now lift this object while imagining how every cell in the body contributes to the lift. Cells may be tiny, but altogether, they create us. Now notice how the weight feels lighter when the lift is accompanied by such a global cellular focus.

Cytoskeleton Music

In this imagery exercise, we boost the cytoskeleton's musical potential. Imagine that the filaments react to movement. Visualize the filaments as the strings of an instrument, such as a violin or a guitar. After every step you take, the filaments vibrate. This vibration causes the cell membrane and all organelles to relax.

Now choose an area of the body to fully exemplify this image. The lower back would certainly be grateful for more musical inspiration. Move your back and imagine that the tubules and filaments of the cells in the lower back are vibrating like strings. Perhaps you can think of a string orchestra or a group of guitars. Imagine the cellular musicality expanding all over the cytoplasm, the membrane, and, eventually, the entire cell. Enjoy the sense of vibration deep in your cells.

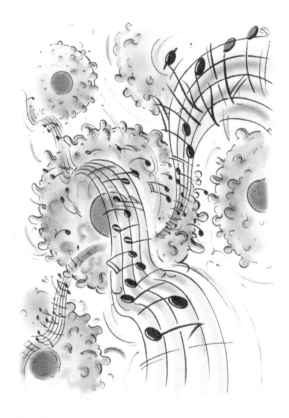

Illustration 32. Cytoskeletal musicality

The Cell Nucleus

The nucleus is the cell's biggest organelle, and it contains deoxyri-bonucleic acid (DNA), your individual genetic information. Thus, the nucleus can be regarded as the cell's library and copy shop. It is here that the blueprint for everything the body can create is stored. If needed, these plans are copied and sent along to the production sites in the ribosomes within the cells. Some parts may be created in the cell's matrix, just outside the cell.

The nucleus's size and location vary depending on the type of cell. Some cells consist almost solely of the nucleus, with the other organelles pushed to the edge. Liver cells have two nuclei because their diverse metabolic processes need several "brains." In a muscle cell, the nucleus is located on the edge so it doesn't block the contraction process. Cell nuclei can swell or shrink, depending on outside stressors. In this sense, the nucleus is "trainable" like a muscle. Stress, aging, and diet also affect the nucleus's size.

The nucleus is wrapped in a double-walled membrane, which tem-porarily dissolves during cell division. The membrane is supported by a framework of intermediate filaments, on both the inside and outside. On the outer membrane, ribosomes dangle like ripe fruit. They con-stantly work to provide the inner and outer coat with spare-part pro-teins.

In several places, the coat is fused together and forms little pores that look like small oval windows. The nucleus communicates with the cyto-plasm through these pores. One can imagine one of these pores to look like three piled-up tires. An elastic basket hangs from the innermost tire into the central space of the cell's nucleus. This basket looks like a bas-ketball hoop and deforms itself respectively as "molecule balls" pass by. The two proteins called exportin and importin organize the selection of molecules passing. Smaller proteins can float through unrestrictedly.

The cell's intelligence also lives in the cytoplasm. If a nucleus is planted into a different cell, the foreign nucleus begins sending out instructions that suit the new cytoplasm's requirements. Thus, the relationship between nucleus and cytoplasm isn't one-sided and hierarchical; the plasma also informs the nucleus, just like your senses inform your brain.

Cell Membrane, Nuclear Membrane: Looking In and Looking Out

Imagine yourself sitting on top of the nuclear membrane, looking inside. What would you see? Imagine yourself sitting on top of the cell membrane, looking inside. What would you see in there? Then imagine yourself sitting on top of the cell membrane, looking outside. What might you see? Imagine yourself sitting on top of the nuclear membrane and looking out. What do you see?

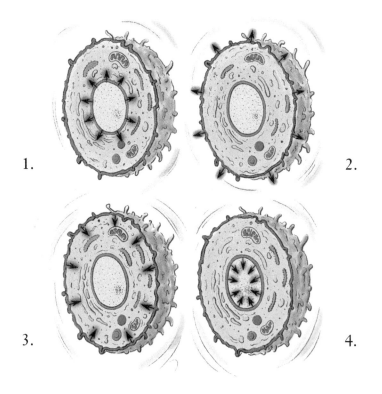

Illustration 33. Looking in and looking out (see exercise above)
1.   Looking outside in from the nuclear membrane
2.   Looking outside in from the cell membrane
3.   Looking inside from the cell membrane
4.   Looking inside from the nuclear membrane

The Chromatin

DNA is a molecule that encodes the development and function of not only human beings but of all life, as we know it. In other words, DNA as a molecule is ancient; it has been around from the dawn of life. This genetic material lives in the nucleus in the form of chromosomes, which are segmented and are clearly visible under a microscope. The DNA in chromosomes is tightly wound, or it would not fit in the cell. If you would stretch out the DNA in your chromosomes and line it up, you would have a strand about six feet long.

Chromosomes are also important for accurate copying of the DNA during cell division. During the intermediate cell-division phase, the chromosomes unroll themselves and unfold into long threads. In this state, the genetic information is called chromatin. In cell division, the chromatin is yet again rolled up tightly like a braid so the genetic code can split easily and so no DNA thread is lost in one of the cell's corners. The chromatin thread's ends are attached to the interior wall of the nuclear wall. We can imagine the chromatin looking like a chain of light bulbs, festoons, or gems stretched out between two spots on the nuclear wall like during a garden party.

Chromosomes as Flexible Fluorescent Pipes

Visualize a very special area in the middle of the cell: the nucleus with the genetic code consisting of chromosomes. Imagine that your chromosomes are emitting bright light. They look like flexible fluorescent pipes floating in a substance. If a chromosome doesn't want to brighten, no need to worry as it also occasionally happens with fluorescent lights. When you revisit them, these chromosomes will be bright and shiny.

Now observe how small beads, which are messages from the nucleus in the form of ribonucleic acid, RNA, are floating past to encounter the ribosomes. Together, the RNA and ribosomes will produce proteins, therefore creating your substance. Thus, you can observe how you are being created. Imagine the ribosomes and RNA sparkling like little stars.

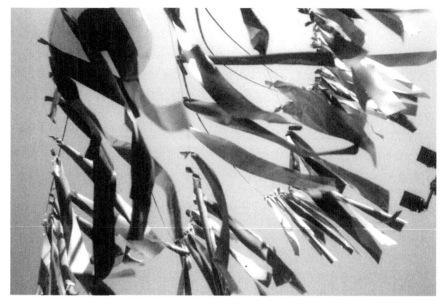

Illustration 34. Chromosomes as fluttering flags

Cellular Nutrition

Imagine a delicate white powder being deposited onto the chromosomes. This white substance melts into the chromosomes. Imagine the powder as the ideal diet for the nucleus. You immediately feel a wondrous effect on your cells, as well-being and energy spread throughout your entire body.

The Genes

The complete set of genes encoded in the DNA and located in the nucleus of the cell is called the genome. The word *genome* is derived from the genes, which represent the cell's blueprints for building your physical structure. In any given cell, only those genes that match the cell's function will be active. In a liver cell, for example, the liver-typical genes are active, whereas in the muscle cell, those genes are active that support muscle function. Myogenin for example, is the key gene in muscle building. If one were to plant it into a non-muscle cell, for example a into cartilage cell, the cell would begin to build muscle cells.

All of your body's cells contain the same genes. If all cells have the same blueprints for proteins, why do we consist of different types of tissue instead of just one? This is because not all genes within a cell are switched on. Let's go back to the image of the cell nucleus as a library. Which blueprints are being selected for copying and turned into proteins strongly depends on the cell's environment and, most of all, on the cell nucleus's surrounding cytoplasm. Your movement and mental behavior in general also affect this process. The genes are not just on autopilot; they also listen to their surroundings and to the actions of the whole person and respond accordingly.

If one were to plant the nucleus of a frog's skin cell into the frog's egg cell, skin would stop building up because those genes would now be receiving egg cell signals from the surrounding cytoplasm, which activate the genes to create a complete frog. The gene would actively change from the building of skin components to the needs of the egg cell because the genes are now in the cytoplasmic environment of the egg cell. This experiment demonstrates that all cells contain the same genes and that the cells' environment activates genes.

In humans, the genome consists of 46 chromosomes, or 23 chromosome pairs. In each of these chromosome pairs, one chromosome comes from the mother and the other from the father. Only one pair, the sex chromosomes, determines the gender. The remaining 22 chromosomes are called autosomes.

Messages for the Nucleus

Focus on the nuclei of your cells. Feel how they are connected to the entire cell, and with the whole body. Formulate positive self-talk, a nucleus mantra, to help your genes send out the most positive instructions: for example, "The genes in my cells send out positive, perfect, and joyful instructions to make my body healthy and strong."

The Double Helix

The DNA is structured in the shape of the famous double helix, which is a double spiral wrapped around an imaginary axis. This shape enables the packing of a lot of information into a small space and facilitates the copying of instructions, called transcription. This copying process is essential to the production of proteins and thus is a very delicate procedure. The copying takes place with the help of RNA, which takes the gene's information, leaves the nucleus through the cell pores, and travels into the cytoplasm.

If the blueprint is copied incorrectly, protein deformations may develop that can be harmful for the body. Naturally, the nucleus has built-in controls, but sometimes even these fail, often under the influence of environmental pollution and harmful rays of sunlight.

Segmentation

The nucleus's so-called working phase is the time in which lots of copying is being done to build new proteins and other substances. During cell division, the copying is stopped and the cell is fully engaged with the division process. The segmentation is also called mitosis, though the halving of the chromosome number, which is necessary in the correct segmentation for the production of sperm or egg cells, is called meiosis.

The interphase is significantly longer than mitosis. Mitosis occurs "automatically" to maintain the cell's youthfulness, but it can also be influenced by movement behavior. If you exercise a lot, you will be producing more cells in the brain's hippocampus, which is important for the relaxation response and for memory. Certain cells cannot reproduce, whereas others do so constantly. For example, the cells in the lining of your gut are always reproducing; you basically have a new lining every day. This is a good image, if you have a sense of humor. You can justifiably say, "Every day, I am a brand-new person in the lining of my intestines." You are also producing a lot of cells in your red bone marrow, about a million or more every second. You are basically a cell millionaire when it comes to new arrivals, which happens every second of your life. This is quite an exciting thought, and one that helps us to appreciate abundance in life. We are always abundant in blood-cell production, even if our bank accounts have momentary lows.

Injuries and cell death are further reasons for the body to speed along mitosis. Danger looms when mitosis becomes uncontrollable. This process of uncontrolled mitosis is known as cancer. Uncontrolled spreading through the tissues is another unpleasant ability of cancer cells. Luckily, the cell has various controls that attentively watch over cell growth, DNA synthesis, and the correct organization of chromosomes.

Cell division is broken into five phases: prophase, prometaphase, cytokinesis, telophase, and anaphase. In prophase, the nucleus disappears and the chromatin condenses into chromosomes. The function of chromatin is to organize DNA into smaller packages, help with mitosis, prevent DNA damage, and help control DNA replication and how a gene expresses itself. In prometaphase, the nuclear coat disappears and the freshly doubled chromosomes begin aligning themselves along the equator of the spindle-shaped cell. In anaphase, the chromosomes travel to the pole of the cell opposite of where they started. The cell then literally zips itself up along its midline. In telophase, the nucleus is newly formed and the chromosomes become more loosely wound. Cytokenesis takes care of the cell plasma's equal distribution with the rest of the organelles.

Experience Chromatin's Resonance

Imagine the chromatin floating in the nucleus. Feel how it is positively affecting the nuclear fluid and contents of the nucleus. You can compare this function to tea leaves changing the water in which they are floating. The tea creates a pleasant vibration in the water. Imagine how this vibration spreads a positive and constructive energy all over the body. Imagine that your DNA's repair mechanisms are functioning perfectly and that at every stage of your cells, all is proceeding smoothly and elegantly.

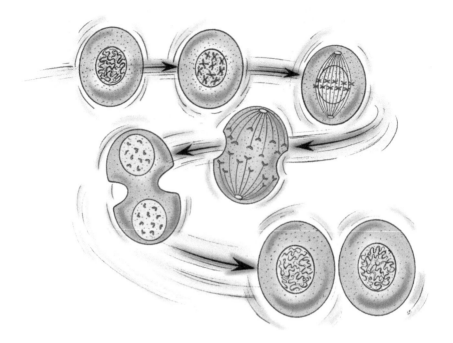

Illustration 35. The process of cell division

Chromosomes Are Prayer Scrolls

This next exercise you may want to try is based on an inspiration from Buddhist practices. You do not need to be a Buddhist to benefit from imagined prayer. In fact, prayer has been shown to have numerous health benefits. If you prefer to simply use the words *self-talk* and *mental imagery* instead of the word *prayer*, feel free to do so.

In Tibetan monasteries, you can find rows of wheels that you spin with a push of your hands as you walk past. The spinning of these wheels on their poles activates the prayers on the scrolls. The activating of the scrolls while passing by appears to me as a type of moving prayer.

I imagined the chromosomes in my nucleus to be like a prayer scroll. My inhalation and exhalation were the hands that spin the scrolls. Although these prayers were not formulated specifically in words, I could feel their positive effects all over my body as an inner cleansing and healing.

Feel free to alter the imagery in any way that suits you, as personalization is always excellent for impactful imagery. You could also imagine that your breathing lights up the chromosomes and bathes them in healing energy. The main thing is to generate a positive feeling for your DNA and the contents of the nucleus.

Mitosis Stretching

Now let's work on some stretching. Lift your arms up over your head or flex and extend your back—try anything you want that will provide the experience of a stretch. Imagine that you are currently supporting cellular activity. Your movement will begin to switch on certain genes in the nucleus that will transcribe proteins to support what we are doing. Initially, this may seem like an outlandish thought, but it is true. My movement influences gene expression and which genes are being switched on.

We know that people with osteoporosis, a thinning of the bone, need to move a lot and to put weight on the bones. This helps stimulate the genes in the bone cells to create more bone tissue. Simply move your body for just 30 seconds with this astonishing image in mind. You are creating your body at all times by how you move and do not move.

Science and Imagery: Healthy Cell Division

Cancer is a complex disease. The following instruction should certainly not be regarded as complete but rather as a beginning of the work needed in this area. Many factors act on the mental, emotional, tissue, and cellular level to prevent the development of cancerous cells. Some respectable scientists say that, depending on the type of cancer, there is nothing you can do to prevent it, as the body is basically on a negative and automatic program that cannot be stopped by imagery. Others, such as Larry Dossey, have analyzed the scientific evidence on the effects of prayer and found some encouraging results (Dossey, 1995).

Even though I am a dedicated mental imagery teacher, I am not stating here that imagery can heal everything. I advise you to seek the best medical help you can. In the future when we have developed our mental powers to a much greater degree, it may be possible to surmount the most challenging diseases with imagery, prayer, and affirmation. Many people claim to have been healed in this fashion, yet for the science-minded, these claims are anecdotal and not evidence-based. In contrast, scientific studies with positive results are about twice as likely to be published as the studies with negative results, says a recent article in the *New York Times*, so all is not well with evidence, especially when it comes evidence on the use of pharmaceuticals (Goldacre, 2013). At the very least, prayer and positive self-talk will not harm you and will most likely benefit you, and they are free and extremely portable! All they take are you and your focused mind.

Here are a few powerful affirmations to help maintain a positive and focused mind:

- I can process all of my life experiences, good or bad, in a relaxed and confident manner.
- My immune system is strong, I exercise sufficiently, and my diet is healthy and balanced.
- My DNA is strong and resistant. My body checks for healthy cell division and can master any situation.
- My DNA is in fabulous health, and my cells are creating the very best proteins for a healthy body for life.

The Cell Matrix

The cells' outer environment isn't simply an airless space but the extra-cellular matrix, which we have previously described as a garden around the cell. This matrix consists of a gel with fibers. The gel is composed of complex sugars, called polysaccharides, which are swimming in a liquid of mineral salts, nutrients, and waste materials. The fibers can be compared to strings or ropes of collagen. Less abundant is elastin, which, as the name implies, is more like a rubber band than the inelastic and strong collagen. One can imagine the matrix as a type of pudding in which different strings and rubber bands are floating around. This imagery may not sound appetizing, but the composition of this pudding largely determines the existence and thus the function of your tissue.

Generally, there are two types of extracellular matrix. One is located in the connective tissue, and the other in the epithelial tissue. Examples of connective tissue include bones, cartilage, tendons, ligaments, and fascia. Examples of epithelial tissue include the skin as well as the interior walls of the esophagus and the entire digestive tract.

Cells Swimming in the Primordial Ocean

Imagine you are in the space between the cells. This might require a very vivid imagination, but if we come to realize that all living beings are descended from unicellular organisms that lived hundreds of millions of years ago in the primordial sea, this imagery becomes easier to grasp. Your cells are swimming in the primordial sea, which is your matrix. Interestingly, the fluid in your cells remains of a similar composition to that primordial sea from which we originated. You may imagine the collagen strands as floating seaweed, for example.

By floating through this primordial sea, you can reach all of your body's cells. This may provide you with a feeling of inner connectedness. Information is being exchanged through fluid; messengers float past you, dissolved in the water like traces of paint. All cells are in touch with each other via the matrix's liquid. The water gives you warmth and cushioning and also acts as your vehicle, as if you were in a slow-moving body of water to be transported everywhere by a current without any observable shape.

If you would like a metaphor, imagine that you are floating in the matrix, similar to the leaf of a water lily on a pond.

Now without losing this sensation of being in the fluid matrix, perform a movement, such as stretching your arm forward. Imagine that from within, the inner flow is being performed smoothly. Do you want to transfer any aspect of this sensation into everyday life? Perhaps if we sense inner flow, everything in our outer lives will flow with ease as well.

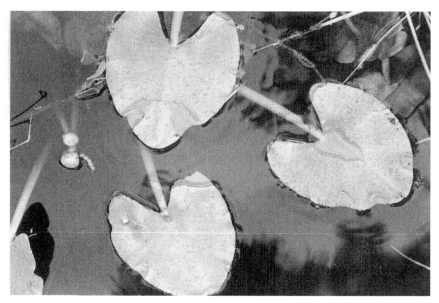

Illustration 36. Cells floating like water lily leaves on a pond

Air Mattresses on the Ocean

Imagine your cells as thousands of small air mattresses swimming in the cell liquid ocean. The cells float on this ocean and can rest on this ocean. The cells are calm and relaxed; there is a holiday kind of feeling in all of the tissues. This sensation allows all tissues to replenish themselves. We can support this state by practicing and repeating this mental formula: "My cells rest and replenish themselves. My cells rest and replenish themselves." This is also a good formula to speak quietly before you go to bed. After you have practiced for a while, notice your state of calmness and enjoy the sensation of cells surrounded by liquid and cells being carried by the water. Can you take this sensation into sitting, standing upright, and walking?

CHAPTER 4

The Skin: A Protective Mantle of Cells

The skin is the body's largest organ. It surrounds us like a protective coat and forms the physical barrier between the rest of the world and us; however, this barrier isn't like a wall and is somewhat permeable and quite sensitive. In the embryo, the skin develops from the same cells as the nervous system, and even in the adult, it is still closely related to the nervous system. The radiation of pain onto the skin due to pressure on the spinal cord nerves is relatively common. Rashes and several skin diseases are sometimes caused by disharmony and stress within the nervous system. Equally, we can positively affect the nervous system through the skin. We all know that a good massage creates a comfortable inner sensation of harmony throughout the body.

Composition, Tasks, and Abilities of the Skin

Your skin, together with your muscles and fascia, forms the biggest sensory organ of your body. Your muscles—or, more precisely, the proprioceptors within the muscles, fascia, ligaments and the tendons—help you experience the speed and dynamics of your movement and in what position your find yourself at any given moment. The skin contains millions of neural end organs, called primary sensory neurons, which can distinguish warmth and cold, strain and pressure, and much more. With the help of our skin, we can perceive movement. If, for example, you bend your elbow, the skin stretches on the outside and creases on the inside. The stretching of sensory organs within the skin informs the brain along with other organs in the muscles and tendons how movement is occurring.

The skin is a hypersensitive radar that can perceive even the smallest changes in the environment, but skin doesn't have the same level of sensitivity all over the body. Its senses are especially acute and sophisticated on the face as well as on the hands and feet. Blind people read with their fingertips and otherwise develop great sensitivity in their skin, which replaces their eyesight. The skin on the back of the hand is relatively unsensitive. Overall, women have better sensibility in their skin than men do, while men have thicker skin, especially on the back.

The skin consists primarily of two layers, called the epidermis and the dermis. The epidermis protects us from water and infection. The dermis houses the sensory organs, sweat glands, and other functional structures. These layers are on top of a thin connective tissue and fatty layer called the superficial fascia. The superficial fascia is also a conductor of nerves and vessels. Below the superficial fascia lies the deep fascia, which rests on the epimysium, the connective-tissue mantle of the muscle. The superficial fascia and fat under your skin appears to be unique to mammals, and it is sometimes claimed to have been an adjustment to spending a lot of time in the water. This fatty layer is particularly pronounced in seals and other water-bound mammals.

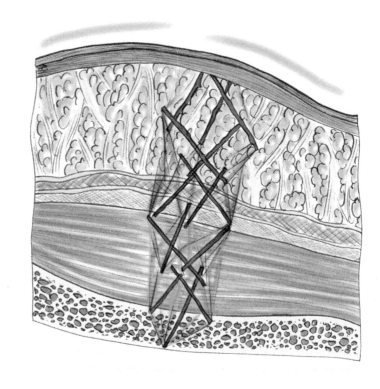

Illustration 37. The layers of the skin and fascia have organization similar to that of tensegrity.

The skin breathes and is also a purifying organ. We can absorb oxygen through the skin and emit toxins as well. Along with the lungs, the intestine, the liver, and the kidneys, the skin is a most important organ in this regard. Unhealthy eating and drinking habits can be reflected in the look of your skin.

The human skin distinguishes itself from animal skin through the almost complete lack of hair. What is perceived as aesthetic in an animal, such as beautiful fur, is unpopular in humans, who generally prefer that hair in any substantial amount be present only on the head, and perhaps in males on the chest and legs as well. How this came to happen along our evolution remains unclear. Does it have advantages in the conservation or reduction of heat? Do we need hair only on the head because we are walking upright? In any case, thanks to the naked skin, fashion—one of humanity's major creative playing fields—emerged.

The skin itself is a complex piece of clothing, which essentially consists of two layers with special features. The outer layer, as previously mentioned, is the relatively thin epidermis, which consists of cells located close to each other, thereby forming a barrier against the penetration of microbes, chemicals, and radiation. Underneath the outer layer lies the tissue-like dermis, which is constructed of scattered cells with a lot of ground substance serving as scaffolding. Both layers contain numerous sensory organs. The epidermis is the product of a cell layer that is located closely above the dermis, called stem cells. These stem cells constantly produce new skin cells, which are pushed to the surface and become increasingly flatter during this process. The reproducing stem cells basically hoist the cells above them to the surface. On the surface, the skin cells die off and form a protective layer of hard, flat cells called the stratum corneum.

The dermis, which is much thicker than the epidermis, consists of collagen fibers, blood and lymph vessels, and flat muscle cells and nerve endings. Macromolecules called glycosaminoglycans in the dermis matrix ensure the presence of water, allowing for the skin's firmness; cosmetics advertise among other things to tighten and hydrate the skin with these substances. The skin also contains elastic and collagen fibers organized in a tensegrity-like fashion, enabling it to return to its original state after a stretch.

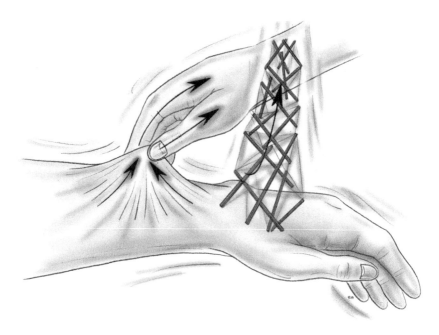

Within the skin there are sweat glands, which are called exocrine glands. Exocrine glands disperse their secretions to the outside of the body, the digestive tube, or the skin, in contrast to the endocrine glands, which channel their products into the bloodstream.

Skin changes throughout the course of life. Children's skin is soft, relatively dry, smooth, and without wrinkles. The glands are barely active yet. During puberty, more hair grows and the skin becomes generally somewhat darker. Aging skin that has been exposed to sun and wind increasingly produces wrinkles, becomes drier, and starts to slacken.

Skin is by nature supplied generously with blood, more than would be necessary for its nourishment alone. This suggests a further function of the skin: It is the body's cooling system. If the air is cold, the vessels in the skin contract to conserve warmth, and if the air is hot or you are exercising intensively, the vessels in the skin relax and the blood can cool as it reaches the surface. The sweat that evaporates from the skin helps in this cooling process.

Skin is also important for maintaining blood pressure. Blood flow can be controlled and directed through selective constriction of the vessel walls. Thus, the blood is channeled either through the skin directly or through many detours, depending on whether the blood pressure is to be increased or lowered. The situation is comparable to a system of sluices, in which the same amount of water can be distributed into more or fewer channels. Holland, specifically Amsterdam, has the macro version of such a system. If the pressure is to be lowered, the gates open and the water is distributed into many channels, making the water level (the blood pressure) go down. If the gates are closed, the water is distributed into fewer channels and the water level (the blood pressure) increases.

The skin contains many lymph vessels, which pervade the skin with a dense network of tiny channels. The lymph vessels don't have any muscular control, and the veins have very little muscle. To achieve good blood circulation, the vessels are dependent on outer influences such as movement, muscle pressure, massage, and warmth. Thus, through exercise, the cleansing of the skin can be stimulated. As with all skin and vascular problems, exercise constitutes one of the most effective therapies. Hot and cold showers are great to exercise the blood vessels. As you take such a shower, focus on the training of you and your vessels at the vascular fitness center.

Your skin color partly depends on circulation, but is mostly determined by the pigment melanin. It is produced by the melanocytes, cells that are equally present in all human races. Whether an individual has dark or light skin is determined by the amount of melanin and the melanosomes, which are small pigment bodies produced by the melanocytes. Tanning isn't an increase of pigment cells, but rather the result of the melanocytes' increased activity. Pigment bodies have the exquisite ability to position themselves on top of the nucleus like a roof, in order to protect it from dangerous ultra-violet rays. These rays can be dangerous for the DNA. Melanin and pigment bodies can also be passed along to neighboring cells so that they as well can be protected from damage.

The epidermis also contains Langerhans cells, named after their German discoverer, Paul Langerhans. For a long time, the function of Langerhans cells was unknown, yet they stood out because of their interesting tennis racket-shaped organelles. Today it has been shown that Langerhans cells have a significant function for the immune system. Thanks to their big exterior surfaces, which are full of receptors, they serve as guardians for the immune system on the body's surface. Intruders can be identified early and the immune system given an early warning.

Inner Wells

One fourth of the liquid available to us daily is produced by the mitochondria as a byproduct in the generation of energy. If you get the chance to sit in a sauna now and then, try to remember the sensation of the sweating and transfer this image to the body's mitochondria. They are literally sweating water in addition to ATP, CO_2, and free radicals.

Now choose an area on your skin that feels dry, rough, or wrinkly, and place your hand on it. Imagine how the mitochondria are producing liquid underneath your hand and how they are distributing this fluid in the tissue. Maintain this image for about a minute.

You can also put your hands on your face and simply imagine fluid populating your skin from the inside out, from whatever the source may be, including drinking pure, clean water. Now take your hands off and you may possibly feel that the area is now softer, smoother, and firmer. This inner "liquid cosmetic" is available to you at any time.

Vitamin D for Cellular Protection

Vitamin D constitutes an important safety factor for the cell membranes. This vitamin is constantly preoccupied with neutralizing antioxidants.

Place your hands on your face or on a different area of your skin. Imagine that you can perceive vitamin D active in the skin. Send uplifting and energizing thoughts to your vitamin D so it can fulfill its tasks thoroughly and persistently. Thus, the cell membrane becomes softer and more flexible, feels smoother, and looks lighter. You can do the same for any other substance important for the skin, including collagen (feel its abundance and strength) or the water-binding glucosaminoglycans.

Stem Cells: The Multitalented Ones

Stem cells are pluripotent cells, a type of ancestral cell. Stem cells create copies of themselves and differentiate into different tissue by cell division. In this fashion they ensure that new tissue is built, without dying themselves. It is quite a stretch of the mind to imagine that the cells in your body are uninterrupted divisions of endless generations of cells from the beginning of life. Obviously, there was no interruption, or you would not exist. Most likely, traces of all who came before us still exist to some degree in our cellular memory.

These days, researchers attempt to transform stem cells into desired tissues. Stem cells from bone marrow in an adult have been converted into nerve cells, for example. Stem cells can adjust themselves to their environment. Metaphorically speaking, they turn into bakers if put in a bakery, or they become carpenters if put into a building site. Stem cells are always the same cell to start with, as they have the potential to take over any task in the body. Once they have taken on a specific task, they stay with it and are unable to convert back again, though someday, I am sure, that trick will also be unraveled by the scientific mind.

Stem Cells Renew Skin

Place your hands on an area of your skin. Imagine that there are constantly new cells being reborn in the epidermis. Send the stem cells power, energy, vitality, beauty, or whatever you would like to achieve so they can pursue the skin's renewal with vigor. Imagine that all damaging influences are being banned.

Nourishment for the Skin

Visualize your dermis and the cells inside it. Imagine that these cells are producing plenty of glycosaminoglycans. They are lovingly attracting and maintaining the water in your skin. Imagine your skin becoming firmer and fuller. Visualize yourself both from the inside and from the outside as you look at your wonderful skin. Sufficient water in the skin's matrix makes the skin feel brighter, lighter, and well nourished. The cells also produce plentiful fibers in order to ensure the skin's youthfulness. The skin is being thoroughly supplied with blood, and the skin cells are well nourished. The skin's immune cells, the Langerhans cells, are awake and energized; the lymph vessels are cleansing the skin from the inside. As you practice vividly generating these sensations and images simultaneously throughout your body, your skin will glow.

The Skin as a Sensory and Emotional Organ

As I mentioned earlier, the skin is a sensory organ closely connected with the nervous system. It sends information about your environment and movements to the brain, and, when a rapid reaction is required, it sends the information through the spinal cord to trigger a reflex response. The way we perceive our skin relates greatly to our level of comfort in our bodies. Have you ever thought about your skin in this fashion? Do you like your skin? Dislike it? If you do not like it, do you have plans to work at changing it? Even if you have blemishes, you cannot simply quit your skin like you might quit a job. Your skin is here to stay. It is therefore important to develop a happy relationship with your surrounding, which on the most intimate level is your skin.

Start with dynamic imagery, positive self-talk, and sufficient exercise. Add the occasional massage, steam bath, or rubdown with a soft cloth while taking a shower. The morning is a great time to stimulate your skin in a positive way; morning stimulation may do more for you to feel awake and alert than drinking coffee. When we exercise we commonly focus on the goal or our movement, or muscles that are being trained. Have you ever exercised and focused on the movement of your skin rather than on your muscles? If you start feeling the movement of your skin it may transform the experience you are having and even increase the benefits you get from exercise.

Sensing Your Skin During Exercise

Imagine your skin to be a warm and protective coat. Focus on an area of your body—for example, your right arm. Stretch it out in front of you. Imagine how your skin is resting on the right arm, enveloping the arm. Imagine all the sensory organs in your skin, ready to relay good news to the brain. Move your right arm and imagine how the arm carries the skin and how the skin is being stretched and condensed as you move; feel how the bones and muscles are active beneath the skin. Bend and stretch your elbow and the wrist, and feel the stretching of the skin on the outside and the kinking of the skin on the inside. Experience your skin as a comfortable, movable stocking around your arm. Imagine millions of skin cells enjoying the stimulating motion.

After all of this imagery and movement, compare how both your arms feel. The right arm probably feels more alive, smoother and more flexible. Now repeat this exercise with the left arm.

Initiating Movement in the Skin

We are used to initiating movement from our joints and muscles; however, now is the moment to give your skin a chance to experience the same. First, simply imagine being able to trigger movement through your skin. If the skin on your face wants to turn to the right, you turn your head to the right. If the skin on the face wants to turn to the left, you turn your head to the left. Look up and then down again, as you imagine your skin triggering this movement. Your head willingly obeys your facial skin's desired direction of movement.

Now transfer these sensations to your entire body. If the skin wants to move the arm forward, the arm stretches forward, and if the skin wants to move the leg forward, you take a step. As you entertain these thoughts and images, you may notice that your body's perception is increasing and your whole being feels calmer and more whole.

Now visualize the skin of the shoulder resting softly and warmly on the shoulder muscles. Even just the thought of this lets your shoulder muscles relax themselves. Then imagine how the skin on your back is resting on the back muscles, warm, comfortable, and having some weight. Already, the back muscles are relaxing.

In everyday life, we may formulate the thought, "My skin is a tension monitor and ensures that the muscles always remain efficient and adapted to the situation." If a muscle is tense, the skin can act as if it is providing the body with a massage, and the movement of the skin lets all tension melt away.

The Power of Imagery to Rejuvenate your Skin

Generally, young people usually don't think about aging and believe that their bodies can last forever. If they overwork or strain themselves, this usually doesn't lead to any immediate issues. Their bodies' ability to regenerate remains strong.

Aging-related physical disintegration starts as if preprogrammed in the cells unless one works against this with mental power and physical consciousness. The power of consciousness is strong enough for an individual to look many years younger than the person actually is.

If you slack mentally, it leads to slacking skin. This may sound exaggerated, but the quality of our thoughts really does, slowly but surely, affect our skin. Harmonious, positive, and loving thoughts create balanced, attractive skin and features. Jealousy, envy, and spitefulness have a subtle and distortive effect on the skin and on the whole body. Our primary thoughts and tendencies will slowly engrave themselves in our features as if we were live sculptures. Additionally, the constant fear of not looking as good as one used to look, or of always having to look perfect, creates tension. Trust strengthens the cells; this is a fact one should not underestimate.

Let's throw an imaginary net over all the negative thoughts that have settled down in our cells. This net will catch these negative thoughts

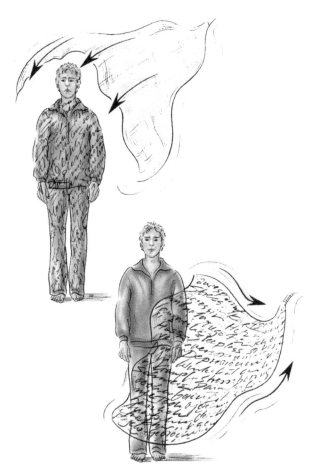

and drag them out of the body. Our bodies are now free from these troublemakers and can replenish themselves with positive thoughts.

Breathing with Your Skin

As humans, we breathe through our lungs but also through our skin. Exhaling through your skin is part of the body's cleansing system and can be supported by regular scrubbing, sauna visits, and mental imagery.

Now imagine that your skin is a giant organ of respiration. As you breathe, feel how the breath moves through the skin, layer by layer. Your inhalation penetrates your body and takes hold of all pollutants, while the exhalation carries these pollutants out of the body. Continuously, with every breath you take, these are being are being eliminated. Practice perceiving the skin on your face breathing. It feels as if the skin is being cleansed. When you are done and feel pure and clean in your skin, you can pull an imaginary protective layer of energy over your skin. This layer will prevent any pollution from getting to your skin.

Collagen Fitness

Collagen is the most common protein in the body. This protein on its own constitutes about 7% of our body weight and is a main product of the connective tissue cells. Collagen is an important constituent of many structures of the body, such as fascia, bone, cartilage, and skin. Without collagen, tissue would be brittle and fragile. Also important to healthy skin is elastin. As is obvious from its name, elastin is very elastic, much more so than collagen. It can be compared to a rubber band. Collagen can be stretched maximally 5%, whereas elastin can be stretched up to 50%. Collagen and elastin are produced in the dermis and help to maintain its structure and smoothness. Aging skin loses collagen and elastin and therefore becomes thinner. The tensegrity of the skin collapses, creating wrinkles, lines, and sagging. Smokers speed up this process and thus often have wrinkles earlier than do nonsmokers.

Collagen Test of the Skin

You can test the elasticity of your skin. Grab some skin on your arm from the area between your thumb and index finger and pull it away from your body (without it hurting). Let go of the skin again, and pay attention to how your skin reacts. If the skin quickly springs back into its initial position, you still have a lot of collagen and elastin; however, if it takes a while to revert, this means that there are somewhat fewer of these proteins present. Be aware that not only this part of your body is elastic but that all connective tissue of your body is supplied generously with these fibers. You can imagine them to be the stretchy, or "tension," part of a tensegrity system. When you pull on your skin, you can imagine that you are stretching such a system, which naturally rebounds to its original shape.

Collagen/Elastin Stretching

Now let's stretch and reach our arms up and to the side. Remember to consciously inhale and exhale. Visualize that many elastic fibers are being stretched and that because of the stretching, the cells are attracting nutrients and creating fresh collagen and elastin, and the movement cleanses your skin. Stretch your body elastically in a variety of directions and imagine your whole body being cleansed and rejuvenated.

Now move your face and feel its elasticity. Make funny faces, and then let them go and feel how your face quickly reverts to its "normal" shape. Practice this several times, until you get a good sense for the facial skin's elasticity.

Take a walk around the room or an outdoor space, if available. Imagine your skin responding to your movement; imagine the muscles and their connective tissue being elastic. Even our bones consist of a lot of collagen; imagine them to be elastic. Notice the effect on your gait; do you feel lighter and springier as you walk?

Exercising Your Collagen with a Partner

We all have heard the phrase "use it or lose it." This phrase is true when it comes to collagen. One of collagen's main tasks is to ensure tissue's resistance to overstretching or sagging. Through conscious and controlled stretching of the tissue, the production of collagen and elastin can be increased and the fluid that resides in the connective tissue circulated. For the following exercise, you will need a partner.

Put one hand on your partner's shoulder while holding your partner's wrist with your other hand. Now gently pull your partner's arm with a focus on elasticity; it's about feeling the elasticity in the arm and amplifying this sensation. The stretch should be gentle and continuous, in no case jerky or too strong. Now, release the arm and begin with a new stretch. Visualize the many elastic strands, the collagen and elastin, coming alive. After several alternations of stretching and relaxing, let your partner compare the sensation, the flexibility and elasticity between arms.

Stimulating Collagen

This next exercise is performed in the upright position. Position your feet parallel to each other and at about hip width apart. Slowly flex your head and then the upper, middle, and lower part of the spine forward. Imagine you are bending one vertebra after the other. Notice the pull of gravity on your head and upper body. Imagine that the stretch in your back is stimulating the collagen and elastin. The elasticity of these proteins is now living its full potential. Imagine that the back is more and more supported by these elastic tissues. The muscles are helping as well, but leave the biggest part of the task to the connective tissue.

Now lift your spine up again by first lifting the pelvis, then the lower, middle, and upper back. Imagine that you are being lifted up by the elastic pull of the collagen and elastin fibers. Finally, your head is balanced precisely over the upright spine.

Repeat the exercise two to three times, focusing on the elasticity and support of the collagen and elastin. Notice how you feel after the last round. Has your posture changed? Can you feel the increased feeling of flexibility in your back?

Firm, Cellulite-Free Skin

Fat has a bad reputation for many reasons. Fat is contained in fat cells, or adipocytes. Fat has gotten its bad reputation from, among other things, cellulite, also called orange peel syndrome. Imagine that you were a fat cell; with such a reputation you would feel rejected and depressed, not the basis of good function. As soon as you start having a more positive relationship with your fat cells, they will be much more willing to change and adapt and become a beautiful part of a harmonious body.

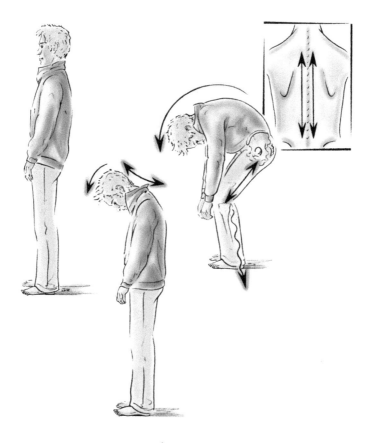

Illustration 40. Rolling down and back up to enliven your collagen

The causes of cellulite are said to be physiological, hormonally related to stress and diet; however, cellulite responds rather poorly to treatments and dietary changes. Genetics are a factor, but the function of genes is very much influenced by the environment, which consists to a great degree of your emotions, mental images, and thoughts. That is why we are going to use mental imagery and address our adipocytes directly.

Imagine that your cells' fat metabolism (lipometabolism) is healthy and balanced, and your adipocytes are doing their very best to please your aesthetic expectations. Now visualize your skin exactly how you wish it to be, providing your cells with a mental model of what you want them to look like, creating beautiful, firm, and balanced skin.

I suggest making a clear decision to walk instead of drive whenever possible. When we walk, we can visualize that our tissues are being cleansed and that all fluid congestion is disappearing. As we use our imagery with conviction, our tissues become stronger and more elastic, thereby supporting firmer skin. We truly become what we are thinking.

Another area of the body that tends to have a rather negative image is the intervertebral disc. Whenever the word *disc* is mentioned, most people instantly associate this with pain, slipped discs, and tight, uncomfortable backs. As with fat cells, an important part of resolving this issue is starting to have a positive image of your discs. It is surprising that most people will readily accept that you cannot achieve a goal unless you formulate it positively, state it, and write it out on a piece of paper. However, when it comes to the body, goals are commonly not formulated at all or are formulated in the negative. Simply ask someone about his or her goal or ideal positive image for the discs and body fat and you will most likely receive a look of disbelief, or even be laughed at. Contrast this reaction to what you will likely get if you ask someone about his or her favorite vacation spot, food place, car, or clothing store. Vacations arouse positive emotions, as does delicious food or perhaps a sporty car. In contrast, strong elastic discs and healthy, happy fat cells sound strange and slightly odd to most people.

"You get what you see" is the main principal of visualization, which has been shown over and over to be scientific fact. If you visualize in the negative, you will find yourself on the path to strange and odd fat cells, in the form of cellulite, and weak discs manifesting as back pain. It is therefore absolutely essential to provide your cells with positive imagery. You are your cells, after all. Don't you want to give yourself a positive lift?

Toning Your Hair

Hair is produced in the epidermis and consists of keratin. It is about .05 millimeters thick and can get as long as a full meter. Evidently, there are even people with hair much longer than that. Hair symbolizes age and social affiliation, and hairstyles change seasonally just as fashion does. If we take a look at pictures that are only 10 to 20 years old, we will notice a very different cultural approach to "hair appreciation" and "hair philosophy" from our own.

A hair consists of a root, a stem, and a muscle that can erect the hair (arrector pili). Hair is produced within the hair follicle. Here, the matrix cells can be found, which reproduce themselves and make the hair grow. These cells need to be active and healthy for the hair to grow sufficiently.

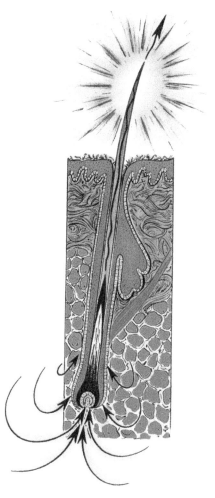

Illustration 41. The roots of your hair are strong and active.

From Wish to Reality

Imagine how the matrix cells divide plentifully (mitosis) and that through this process of division, beautiful and strong hair is created. Mentally whisper to your hair's root cells that they may remain active for many more years or that they may reactivate joyfully if they have slackened in any way.

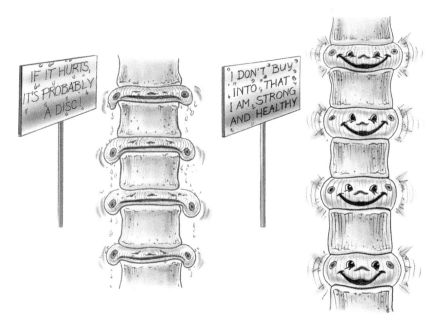

Illustration 42. Turning the intervertebral discs' negative image into a positive image

CHAPTER 5

The Face: Reflection of Cellular Health

You may have noticed that some people who are very handsome at some point in their lives lose their good looks fairly quickly, while others do not change much over time, sometimes over decades. Surely, genetics, diet, exercise level, and the environment affect the way someone looks; however, many new studies are demonstrating that our emotions and thoughts strongly influence our physical state.

The Face and Our Attitudes

In one of those studies, 122 males were asked whether their reaction to their first heart attack was positive or negative. It turned out that the men's attitudes were better predictors of their life expectancy than were their medical factors such as cardiac defect, arteriosclerosis, cholesterol level, or blood pressure. Out of the 25 most pessimistic males, all had died within eight years, whereas among the optimistic ones, only six had died! Thus, mental state was the most prominent indicator for an individual's health (Goleman, 1991).

Stress will surely have an adverse effect on the skin of your face as you furrow your brows and practice a worried and rushed look. This is similar to muscle training; the way your skin is moved and adjusted over time also trains your skin into these positions as the subcutaneous connective tissue remembers the lines of pull, folds, and wrinkles. This type of connective tissue, the superficial fascia, adjusts rapidly and is rather good at remembering what you have practiced. Exercise, including the way you move your facial muscles, makes you better at what you are practicing, even if things are going in the wrong direction. In other words, you do not get what you want but what you practice, so align your practice with what you want.

Posture is a classic example of this. Posture is a lifetime practice and is one of the things you can improve fastest to make yourself look more youthful. A hunched spine, called flexion of the thoracic spine (spine in the ribcage area), is certainly not an attractive or healthy posture. However, in daily life most people practice this a lot more than the opposite, which is spinal extension in the thoracic spine.

When someone feels comfortable in his or her body and has a lot of energy and a positive attitude, this will reflect positively in the person's facial expression. Accordingly, a person's social environment can also have a positive effect on his or her health. In a study of 100 patients who were about to have a bone marrow transplant, 54% of the patients who reported having plenty of support from friends and family were still alive two years later Goleman, 1991). Of the people who said they had little emotional support, only 20% were still alive. Figuratively speaking, the first group "bathed" in a more positive thought environment while, unfortunately, the other group lacked this bath of positive influence.

The good news is that even if we do not have people around us constantly wishing us well, we can still create this atmosphere on our own. After all, we are the producers of our own thoughts.

If the majority of our thoughts are benevolent and constructive, to both others and ourselves, eventually they will start to engrain themselves in our facial features and our bodies. The ancient Greeks said that it was important for a mother to be surrounded by beautiful statues and paintings because this would influence the looks of the unborn baby. The same is true for our own faces. If we surround ourselves with positive thoughts and imagery, this will have a healing and balancing effect on our skins and bodies overall.

Meditations for the Face

Let's imagine the different tissue layers of the face. First is the top layer, called the epidermis, with densely aligned cells forming a waterproof barrier. Below that we find the dermis, with fairly tough connective tissue, sweat glands, and hair follicles. The deepest skin tissue, also called hypodermis, is made of loose connective tissue (superficial fascia) and a thin layer of fat. The superficial fascia in the skin is masterful at adjusting to all the movements of the face. Finally, we arrive at the muscles, which are covered by a different type of connective tissue called the epimysium.

Feel all these layers gently rest on top of each other. Feel how the muscles support the tissues above and how the dermis supports the epidermis. Inhale and imagine your breath moving through all these layers. Exhale and imagine your exhalation purifying all the layers. Inhale again and imagine your inhalation rejuvenating all layers of your skin. Exhale and imagine the layers becoming increasingly smooth and relaxed. Take several more breaths while using this imagery.

The facial musculature is tied to your emotional state via the autonomic nervous system. If you are relaxed and well rested, it will show on your face. Similarly, when you relax your face, this has a regenerative effect on the entire nervous system. Special face massages are used in the practice of Indian Ayurvedic medicine with the goal of influencing the state of the entire nervous system. In the West, different methods of massage are also used for this purpose.

Now let's imagine that all of these layers are communicating with each other. This communication helps to keep the face elastic and relaxed while maintaining its surface tension. Imagine the dynamic nature of the collagen tissue in your skin providing an ideal level of tension. The superficial connective tissue is organized in a tensegrity architecture, which allows the connective tissue in your skin to have a rebounding elasticity.

Imagine your eyelids and the skin surrounding the eyes. The plentitude and dynamics of the collagen and elastin are particularly important. Imagine a lot of space and openness around your eyes. Focus on the skin around the lips and inside the lip muscle itself called orbicularis oris. Stress often manifests through a subtle subconscious tensioning of the muscles and connective tissue around the mouth. For this area to remain smooth, imagine the elastic and resilient power of collagen and the facial muscles. Above all, imagine your lips relaxing, calming down. Create a feeling of soft flexibility in your lips.

Aerobics for the Skin

Exercises that are done for the face without deliberate awareness of the skin aren't very effective and may even lead to more wrinkles. Actions such as tightening and relaxing muscles of your face in specific areas are good if you can feel what you are actually doing. Remember that practice does not make perfect. Practice makes permanent, so if your practice does not contain the mental accompaniment that contains the goals you want to achieve, it may not help to achieve your goals. In fact, we are doing facial exercises all day as we talk and communicate. A first important step is to feel your face moving during your daily activities and see if you are creating tension in your face. At the outset, it may appear to be very odd to be focused on your face when you talk to someone, but it's a great way to discover if you are keeping your face tension-free during the day.

The first step in doing any exercise for your face is to relax your face. Tight muscles and connective tissue reduce your ability to feel what you are doing. The quality of the exercise determines its effectiveness.

Let's start our practice by moving the mouth in a variety of directions. Gently squeeze your lips and then relax them. Repeat this action three times. Lift up the corners of your mouth and then lower them again. Repeat this three times as well. Open your eyes wide and then squeeze them shut. Again, three repetitions are good. Notice how smoothly you can do these movements. You should not just go straight from a position of wide-open eyes to the eyes being shut. There should be plenty of transition between the two extremes.

As you practice, imagine the cells in your skin and connective tissue smiling.
Similarly to the mouth, circular constrictor muscles surround the eyes. Notice that the imagery contained in the anatomical name is not what we want to focus on. Being constricted is probably not our best embod-

iment. If these muscles are tight, you will be practicing wrinkled skin and a worried look.

Imagine the muscles around both eyes expanding like water rings on the surface of a lake. Muscles around the mouth are also expanding. Imagine all of the circular muscles around the eyes and the mouth widening and relaxing at the same time.

Face Lifting, the Natural Way

Wash your hands if you like. Rub them together for a moment to create some warmth and place them on your face, fingers pointing more or less upward. Try to cover as much of your face as possible. Your head should be inclined forward slightly.

Imagine that your hands are supporting the skin you are currently touching. Imagine your skin relaxing in your hands. Focus on the feeling of support provided by your hands, as if the skin, connective tissue, and muscles of your face finally have a chance to let go of all their accumulated tension, dropping it into your hands.

Imagine your hands being sponges for this tension, absorbing it out of your face. Now remove your hands and shake them to release this tension into the environment, where it can be recycled into comfort and well-being. Repeat this process at least three times.

Visualize the skin's cells being cleansed and rinsed thoroughly with fresh spring water. Feel how the cells are being buoyed upward thanks to the connective tissue and skin adapting and restructuring. Imagine them to have sufficient space and spring.

Now imagine that the skin you are touching is actually floating upward. The collagen and elastin are becoming firmer and more buoyant and are pulling every single facial cell upward. The traces that gravity may have left over many years are being erased.

Now remove your hands and feel your new and cost-efficient facelift!

Chi Gong for the Face

In the eastern methods of Chi Gong and Tai Chi, physical health is achieved through energetic consciousness and smooth, coordinated movement. Let's exercise our facial skin and connective tissue while keeping these concepts in mind.

Imagine soothing music, such as flutes, violins, maybe even a harp. Then slowly begin moving your facial skin. This is not set movement. See what is possible for you in the moment, what you feel like doing, as long as it is slow. Sense all the muscles in your face and how they can contract and let go. Move your lips, extend your mouth, and move your cheeks inward and outward. Imagine that your facial skin, connective tissue, and muscles are performing a slow-motion dance. Imagine this dance exhilarating the cells of your face and putting them in a vibrant mood!

Sensitive Skin for the Face

Now move your head in different directions. Look up and down and to the side, and laterally tilt your head as well. Feel how the skin's millions of cells are being carried along with this movement. Imagine the cells of the skin being sensitive to this movement. They perceive every change in position, every turn and twist.

As you move your head, your face is moving through space and through the air. Slowly walk around your room or the area you are in and imagine that the air brushing past your face is massaging and toning your skin. Imagine that all stress is being released from your face.

The Modiolus

The modiolus is a small but significant muscle of the face; it is a junction, the face's navel, so to speak. Just like a wheel hub, the modiolus is a connecting point for many muscles of the face. Tension in the modiolus has an effect on the whole face.

The easiest way to locate the modiolus is to grab the cheek between thumb and index finger about one inch to the side of corner of the mouth. This point may feel somewhat thicker than the rest of the cheek. Gently massage this point between your fingers. Let your fingertips rotate around this point and you may notice that your shoulders and neck are relaxing as well.

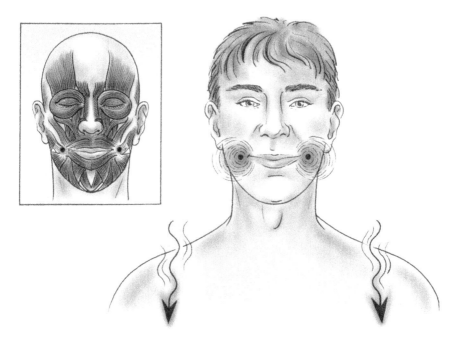

Illustration 43. The modiolus is a central hub of the facial muscles.

As the Hand, So the Face

The degree of tension in the hands is closely related to that of the face. Observe the tension in your facial musculature as you move your hands, paying special attention to the tongue, as well as the constrictor muscles around the eyes and the mouth. As you stretch, contract, and move your fingers in the exercise below, observe any reaction in the muscles of your face.

Make tight fists, stretch out your hand, and shake and wiggle your fingers while observing your face. Hold your right wrist with your left hand and shake it loosely. Imagine that the hand's bones, especially the carpal bones, are small jingling bells. After about a minute, let go and feel how the face and shoulders are more relaxed on the right side. Now repeat the exercise on the left side.

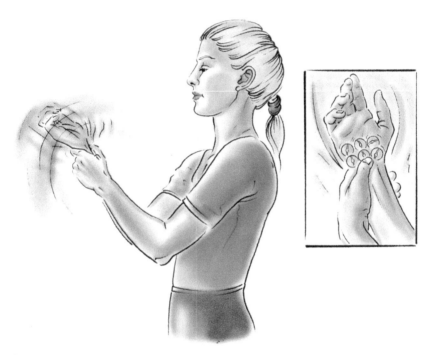

Illustration 44. Relaxing the hands and wrists to help relax the face

Put an End to Headaches with Loving Touch

Headaches certainly do not contribute to a happy and relaxed face. If one suffers from headaches often, even the slightest onset of a headache is enough to alter the face. I would like to share with you a personal experience I've had relative to this important topic.

One time, I was on a ship and I got a very strong headache. I tried several visualization methods, unsuccessfully, and felt pretty disappointed;

however, I knew that every time something like that happened, I would usually learn something new from the experience. As I was suffering from the increasing pain, I told myself that I was ready to learn whatever I had to; it had just better happen fast. Learning something is more easily done while feeling physically well. In previous situations like this, I had noticed that turning off the negative thinking such as "why me" self-talk and instead turning up the positive outlook might trigger the recovery process.

I recalled the relationship between movement and touch. The love of movement can be conveyed via the hands. By feeling a deep reverence, admiration, and love toward the tissue, applying touch to aching areas can bring a lot of relief. Hence, I imagined activating the vibration of love, the feeling of love in my hands, and placed them on my head. Instantly, the pain started to fade. Specific areas were still resisting, however. I simply poured more love over them. When the embodiment of love had settled within every single cell and love's vibration had neutralized the pain's vibration, the headache disappeared within minutes. I realized that in a certain sense, pain is the antimatter, the opposite, of love. Thus, the pain was the stepping-stone to a new insight.

Now, this may sound rather fanciful, but after all, love is an emotion, a feeling that, hopefully, all of us have felt at some time in our lives. If you can remember that feeling and imagine it existing in your hands—or anywhere in your body, for that matter—this is a good start. Results also depend on imagery skills, and these grow with practice. If you read one or two of the exercises in this book every day, you will certainly grow in your ability to generate imagery, maintain it with increasing strength, and modulate it.

Additionally, imagery modulates pain perception and has shown to be helpful to reduce pain in a variety of health conditions (Syrjala et al., 1995). The experience of pain is quite subjective and relates to the perceived outcome after the incidents. Personal beliefs and expectations greatly influence pain levels as well (Bingel et al., 2011).

Imagined pain and actual pain seem to share common pathways. There is evidence that if you think a movement will be painful or not painful, this will influence the performance of the movement (Hugdahl et al., 2001). If you have pain, your movement and muscle activation are altered. Even when the pain is gone, the altered patterns may persist (Hodges, Vleeming, and Fitzgerald, 2010).

Painful emotion and actual pain seem to be processed in the same areas of the brain (Kross et al., 2001). It may be important to be aware of the fact that even a painful emotion will influence movement performance and that it may be useful to develop skills to modulate such imagery. A simple technique is changing your focus to a happy memory. Metaphorical imagery might also help with the pain. First one establishes an image that describes the pain, like pinpricks or something that is red-hot. Then one creates an image that expresses the comfortable state of the same area, such as a smooth and relaxed feeling or a cool blue color. If this is done repeatedly and systematically, it can be very effective.

Breaking through Resistance

A specific area of the body to which one wants to give love will often show resistance. The area will appear as if it doesn't want to accept any of positive feelings being imagined. Also, the tissue may look fuzzy or dark to the inner eye. The painful body part feels confused and dense, not airy and light. This is often the case with injuries. The following exercise may help in this case.

More Light into the Cells

Imagine that in each of your body's cells, a light is being switched on— beautiful candles or another type of illumination brighten the cells. The cells become clearer and translucent. Every angle and every corner of the cells is now being illuminated.

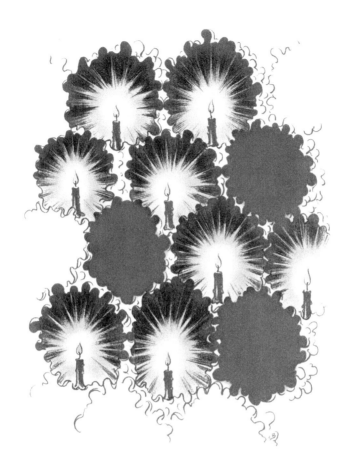

Illustration 45. More light in the cells

Love as the Primal Drive of Movement

Love can be perceived as a vibration, a resonance, or a color, and it can be experienced as a movement in the tissue. The primal drive of every movement is love. If one is happy and satisfied—for example, if one is in love—one feels moved, is excited, and likes to move. The opposite is the case if one is depressed: One feels lethargic and lacks motivation to move.

One doesn't need a partner to feel love; it is not the case that only the perfect soul mate will do the trick. You can also feel love for nature as you stand in front of a beautiful vista, or for art, when you are touched by music or a dazzling piece of visual art. I have seen many performing artists express the love of movement in dance. Have you ever thought of experiencing love for your body's cells in their constant unconditional drive to keep you healthy?

Love Droplets

The following imagery may help you neutralize pain or speed up a healing process.

Imagine you are kneading love into your tissue, as if love were an indispensible component of the very fiber of your body. The love is being blended with your tissue and distributes itself in every area and system of your body: bones and joints, muscles and fascia, organs and nerves.

For those who find it odd to proceed in the way described above, I recommend visualizing the word *love*, perhaps in golden writing. Imagine the word *love* and how the sound of the word resonates. Imagine this sound vibration penetrating your body, dissolving tension points. If sound vibration can shatter glass, then surely it can melt away tension. Pour some droplets of love into the midst of a tense area watch it dissolve into relaxation.

For those who prefer self-talk, it might help to silently enunciate the word *love*. Feel how this sound causes the tissues and cells to vibrate. Imagine the cell membranes, the cytoplasm, and even the nucleus of the cell to vibrate in this positive sound.

CHAPTER 6

The Eyes: Clear Vision with Healthy Cells

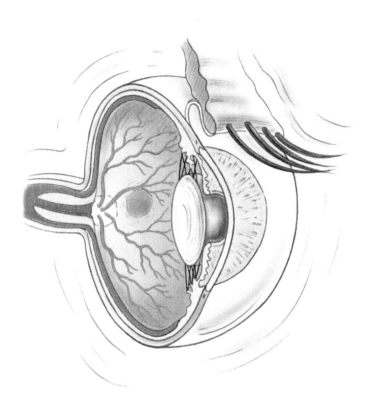

Illustration 46. Anatomy of the eyeball

The eye consists of the eyeball, the muscles moving it, and supporting gadgets such as the eyelids and the tear glands. The eyeball isn't sitting in the eye socket all on its own; it's resting on cushioning fat offering protection and increasing its glide and ability to move (this is another example of positive fat). Examining the eyeball from the outside looking inwards, you can detect that the eyeball itself consists of three layers: the derma, the choroid, and the retina. The retina is the area that actually does the work of receiving light, starting the process of collecting information on what is out there in the wide world around you.

The optic nerve (nervus opticus) enters the eyeball from the back. It consists of one million nerves and sends the collected light information to the brain. Located in the front of the eye is the optical apparatus, including the cornea and the lens. The iris functions as the eye's shutter, if you will, controlling the amount of light allowed in to the pupil. Depending on light exposure, the iris enlarges or minimizes its size with help of a sphincter. The cornea, the lens, and other factors break down the incoming light in order for it to fall onto the retina, where the eye's actual sensory organs, called rods and cones, are located.

A circular sphincter muscle holds up the lens in a manner similar manner to springs supporting the jumping surface of a trampoline. If the sphincter contracts, the lens becomes thicker and slightly smaller. This action allows you to see things close up. If the sphincter relaxes, it becomes wider and the lens gets stretched. In this case, the eye is adjusted for far vision. If you are constantly looking up close, the lens is constantly set to "thick" and the sphincter can get tired. Thus, it is more strenuous for the eye to look close up than to look far off, when the sphincter is relaxed. If the eyes are tired, the face and the rest of the body can also be affected.

Seeing Is Interpreting

In a sense, we see with our brains. The picture that is captured by a healthy eye is relatively diffuse; the brain then edits it to achieve more sharpness and distinctiveness. Thus, it is justified to say that we see with the brain, which is, among other things, an organ that interprets what it perceives. The brain makes the best guess of what it is seeing based on the available data. You may have experienced a time when you briefly saw something along the side of the road that ended up being something completely different from what you originally thought. For example, where you saw an animal, there was really just a bush. For a brief moment, the brain made a guess that turned out to be incorrect. Luckily, most of the time, the brain's assumptions are spot-on. The human brain has, to a certain degree, sacrificed accuracy for speed, often supporting survival. In almost the same manner, we can regard our interior imagery as interpretation: We see everything through lenses colored by our beliefs and expectations. The classic example of this is, once again, love, in which one sees a partner through a rose-colored filter.

Strengthening and Relaxing the Eye Muscles

This exercise both strengthens and relaxes the eyes and the muscles surrounding them. It helps to release tension in the muscles that move the lens and is valuable if you are reading for long periods or if your work involves a lot of time looking at computer screens. Perform this exercise at the office to give your eyes a needed rest. We often can see more clearly after this exercise, including in a figurative sense.

To start the exercise, rub the palms of your hands against each other until they feel slightly warm. Then close your eyes and place your palms on your eyes. Imagine that you are standing on a hill. Located just in front of you is a bush with very attractive flowers. In the distance you can see a leafy tree with clouds above. Focus your vision on the distant tree or on the cloud floating above it. Attempt to see these things as clearly as possible in your imagination. Then allow your gaze to slowly shift to the bushes in front of you. Rest your eyes on the bush and notice the beauty and radiant color of the flowers. You may also smell the flowers while you admire the virtuosity of nature's creation. Allow your gaze to remain there for about half a minute, then slowly shift your gaze back to the distant tree. Imagine that your gaze is resting on the tree, as if your gaze had some weight to it. Now shift your eyes to the fluffy cloud above the tree. The cloud may be moving slowly across the sky, the tree moving with the wind. Repeat this imaginary shifting of your gaze from close up to far away three times. Aim to be effortless throughout. Imagine your eyes resting in their sockets and moving slowly and smoothly.

Now remove your hands from your eyes, which remain closed. Wait for a moment before slowly opening your eyes and sensing the comforting, relaxed sensation around your eyes. Perhaps you even notice that colors have become just slightly brighter, and contours of objects slightly sharper.

Relaxed Neck, Happy Eyes

The state of the neck, including the level of tension in the muscles and the disposition of the fascia, can influence how your eyes feel. How can that be? The cervical spine, with the head balanced on top, is constantly performing subtle adjustments to help the eyes face in the desired direction. If your neck is in an unfavorable position—forward, for example—you are flexing your lower cervical spine while extending your head on top of the spine. This creates a constant state of tension in your neck, and your eyes have a harder time of reaching all their desired facings with ease.

To start the exercise, rest yourself in a supine position on a mat, your bed, or any comfortable surface. Place your hands on your neck, one hand on top of the other. Now imagine that the muscles of your neck are relaxing into your hands. Helped along by the warmth of your hands and gravity, the neck muscles let go of their tension and become softer and wider. If you like metaphors, you may try the idea of the muscles of the neck melting downward like honey dripping from a spoon. Imagine your eyes resting deeply in their sockets. You can possibly combine the two images, the neck melting and the eyes resting in their sockets. Feel how the muscles surrounding the eyes are also relaxing.

This exercise can similarly be performed in a reclined sitting position if you prefer.

Color and Your Eyes

Nowadays, one can purchase contact lenses of any type with color options. That is certainly a way to affect what you see, but how about the inner color, the metaphorical pots of paint that live in the cones and the retina? The rods and cones are the sensory organs, the photosensors of the eye. The black-and-white-sensitive rods are more numerous, numbering about 120 million, and are more sensitive in general, but only the cones can perceive color. The cones come in red-, green-, and blue-detecting varieties. From these colors, all other colors are surmised. Both rods and cones are able to convert incoming light into electrochemical signals, which are subsequently transmitted to the brain.

In the photosensors, the "vision colorants" called photopsins are piled up much like a stack of plates or discs made of pigment. If these color-detecting photopsin discs are used up, they are discarded at the tip of the cell and are recycled. In the following exercise, we are going to support the production and recycling of the color discs.

Replenishing Your Eye Colors

Arrange yourself comfortably in a supine position or in a cozy chair. Close your eyes and place your hands on your face to cover your eyes. Start by imagining the many receptors, the rods and cones, at the back of the eye. Now imagine the color red. See the color red as clearly as possible. Visualize a red rose or a bowl of bright red strawberries. Imagine red is being poured into your photosensors. The cones are being refilled with red.

Now let's try the same thing with the color blue. Visualize a blue sky or a blue ocean, for example—in any case, a vigorous and vibrant blue. This color, blue, is now is filling your cones, which become resplendent with blue.

Next we practice with green. Imagine a green lawn, a green forest, green moss—whatever green you can best visualize. Green, lush and vigorous, is now refilling your cones, a festive green for strong, happy eyes.

Make sure one last time that you have refilled your cones with vibrant red, blue, and green. Then remove your hands slowly. You may notice that you can see colors in your environment more clearly.

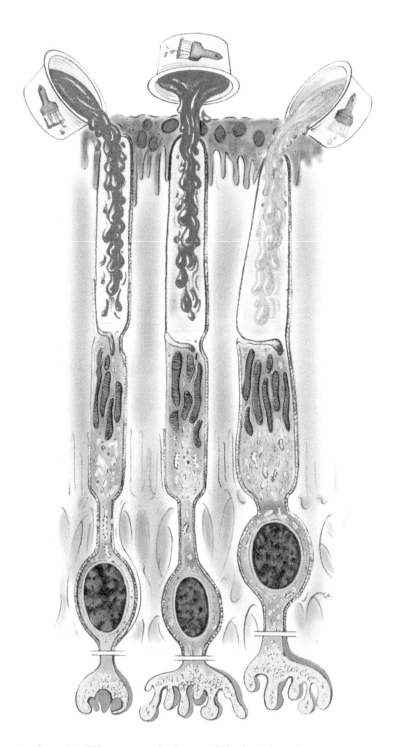

Illustration 47. The cones being refilled with color

CHAPTER 7

Vital Cells: Consequence of Your Behavior

The cells have their own minds, so to speak, and this does not always make sense from a rational point of view. The neurons of the brain, for example, produce what is called noise. Noise consists of messages from the neurons that really do not make any sense from a point of view of getting things done in the brain, at least based on current understanding of the functioning of the brain. It may be that neurons are just happily active, whistling along with their leggy dendrites up, enjoying the view from their vantage point in the brain. The cells' behavioral patterns are based on millions of years of evolution and specific biological events that are well rehearsed. One of these patterns is not good news for your cells. These cells die after a certain amount of time, apparently for no specific reason. In contrast, many cells in your body can live eternally. The gametes represented by the ovum, or egg, in females and the sperm cells in men, as well as stem cells, live forever, at least in a certain sense. These cells divide infinitely and multiply themselves and thus never appear to die. Science is still speculating on why some cells die, but maybe it's best to focus on the cells in your body that potentially have eternal life—if this is to your liking, of course. Interestingly, the metaphorical database and software enabling eternal life are locked somewhere in the secret chambers of your cells.

Science used to postulate that the genes predetermined the structure of human beings to the last very detail; however, the scientists who are dedicated to the mapping of the human genome have discovered that there simply aren't enough genes to predetermine the whole human body. Instead of the expected 100,000 genes, there are in fact only 30,000, which is far too few instructions and blueprints.

The answer to this dilemma is that who we are and what we end up being are influenced by our behavior and environment. *Time* magazine published an interesting article about genetic researcher Craig Venter's work in which Venter states that it's not the genes but the *environment* that is key to our behavior (Ridley, 2003). This new way of looking at the way we end up from a genetic point of view is called epigenetics.

Learning and becoming are thus the selective turning on and off of genes. Our genes are dynamic and adaptable and get their instructions from our behavioral patterns, not just from inherent factors. We are permanently in a dialogue with our genes.

In the West, we often define ourselves according to the newest scientific research, but the changeable nature of our very structural being has long been proposed in Eastern philosophies.

We very much become how we behave, and how we behave is based on the way we move, our posture, our emotions, our mental life, and the predominant imagery and self-talk circulating through our brains. What used to be regarded as so much esoteric hoopla has become the science of the day. Assured by this insight, we can now proceed improve our cellular fitness.

Entering into a Dialogue with Your Cells

How can we enter into dialogue with our cells and genes? How can we deliberately participate in the building of our bodies? Of course we can go to the gym and work out or start repeating some positive words, and so forth. In this book, however, we want to delve a bit deeper and enter into conscious dialogue with our cells, as if we want to hear our cells' voice or opinion, not just our usual mental productions. This will require a bit of calming down and focusing.

Let's imagine the cells have something very positive, flexible, and useful to communicate, while at the same time they have a rather fixed and unchanging nature. If you are a liver cell, a hepatocyte, that is your identity; the same goes for a osteocyte in your the bones, and so on.

Let us say that you can support your cells to gradually change into their most positive embodiments. A hepatocyte for life—well, fine, but what about a super-healthy and fully functioning hepatocyte? Can we possibly transform some of the unyielding aspects of our cells and convince them to behave with more elasticity, variability and ability to absorb positive life energy?

Eliminating What Harms the Cells

First, it is essential to quit doing things that can harm your cells. This means eating healthy, non-processed foods; getting enough activity in fresh air; and getting sufficient exercise. It does not take much to improve fitness; even a 12-minute interval training regimen per day can do the trick. Interval training consists of alternating brief high-intensity workouts with short rest periods. You can even do this using the chair you are sitting on, if it's not of the rotating, unstable, or super-soft kind. For more on how to do this, you can consult my "Sit to Be Fit" program at www.franklinmethod.com).

Overindulgence in negative imagery and self-talk, especially mental activities that increase your stress levels, will be harmful to your cells. This isn't so obvious; you will not get sick immediately, as these things can take a while to manifest. Cellular well-being relies on our habits, both physical and mental. How easy is it to repeat, at this very moment, "I am feeling better with every breath," while thinking, "I feel bad, tense, and tired"? Be careful not say, "I feel great," when you feel pretty awful; that will just feel like lying to yourself. It is often better to evolve your self-talk and imagery incrementally by formulating something such as this: "I am starting to feel better. I am noticing more relaxation in my shoulders. It appears that my breath is deepening now."

The following exercises are designed to absorb health more deeply into your cells. We shall imagine entering into a dialogue with our genes and imagine that we are cleansing our cells, strengthening and motivating them.

Removing Waste from Your Cells

Visualize many tender vacuoles, basically the mini containers and transport pods of the cell. They look like tiny bubbles and float around in the cell. One of the responsibilities of the vacuoles is to transport waste out of the cell. Imagine this process looking somewhat like floating trash bags that move toward the cell wall, where they are dumped out and eliminated. The vacuoles float to the wall of the cell, the double lipid membrane, and fuse with it, and finally, their content is transported through the membrane and ejected. This may feel like letting go of old baggage at the cellular level, a sweeping clean from within the cell of all used-up and stale elements.

Imagine how everything that is dark and negative is removed from the cell and how the cell's insides become sparkling clean. The cell begins to shine from within as if light were radiating from it.

It is almost as if its improved health makes the cell look rosy-cheeked and wearing a happy, liberated impression.

At times, metabolic waste remains in the cell in the form of small granules called lipofuscin granules. Imagine these granules dissolving. Imagine all and any dark spots in your cells getting thinner and then finally dissolving. The cell is now fully cleansed, reminding you perhaps of the feeling you may have after a sauna or steam bath.

Fresh Air for Your Cells

Let us imagine a very large cell in which we have more than enough space to move around. This cell is huge—ballroom- or even cathedral-sized—with many windows. This cell will represent all the cells of your body.

As of this moment, it is a little dark and musty in this cell that is standing in for all your cells. That is why we imagine all the windows opening. (There are plenty, and of course they open magically.) Imagine a refreshing breeze filling the large cell. Sunlight streams into the cellular space and allows for better visibility. We slowly but surely see the colors of the cellular space. If you having difficulty imagining an actual cell, then select a regular room of your liking and imagine it being aired out. Continue with the exercise by imagining the dusty, musty air being replaced with fresh air so that the room or cell feels brighter and cleaner by the moment. It smells and tastes like spring, and there is a sense of all-round rejuvenation in the air. All the windows are open now. A breeze of the perfect temperature and gustiness is blowing through the cellular space, which becomes increasingly brighter and fresher. We can continue to bathe in the sensation of fresh, aerated cells.

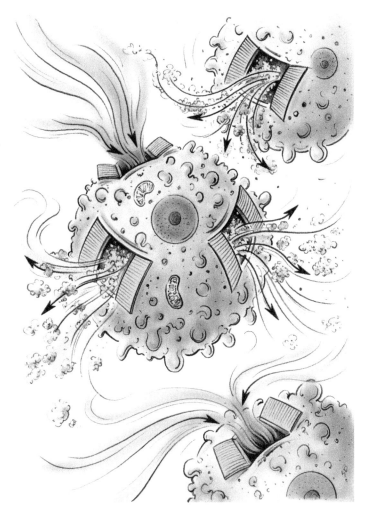

Illustration 48. Imagine opening the windows and filling the cells with clean, refreshing air.

Bright Light Within Your Cells

Similarly to the exercise described above, we can imagine that light is brightening up the cells. Imagine a morning in spring, and bright light streaming into the room through rain-purified air. The cell membranes become more translucent, and light sparkles in the corners and recesses of the cell. The organelles reflect the light and are being bathed in it as well as radiating their own light. See if you can imagine all the cells in the body becoming brighter and fresher. Scan your body and imagine the light becoming brighter everywhere. The brightness is increasing in your torso, spine and pelvis, legs, shoulders and arms, head, and face.

Now imagine a miniature sun that shines brightly and visits every single cell to provide light. Imagine that this sun possesses a healing and cleansing effect.

Use any metaphor that helps you along, such as a lantern or a lampshade being illuminated from within, to imagine light in the cells (see, for example, Illustration 49).

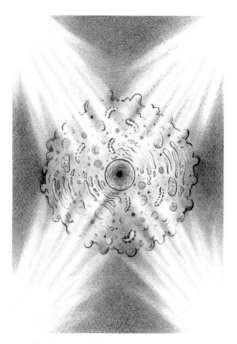

Illustration 49. Bright light illuminates the cells.

The Beauty of Flowers for Your Cells

Have you ever looked at a flower or a bunch of flowers and been affected by their beauty in the sense of thinking, "Wow, that is really a fantastic color and shape"? Many of us have probably experienced wandering through a garden, forest, or some other natural area and feeling refreshed and invigorated thereafter. The garden culture of China and Japan was created for this purpose, as contemplating or walking through a garden can have a mentally and physically balancing effect (Reynolds, 2015). Flowers appear to have a continuously positive attitude; they just stand there and exude beauty. Thanks to flowers, we can indeed charge ourselves with positive energy. Perhaps we can imagine bringing this energy into our cells. The idea of every cell in the body being a flower is perhaps a bit much, but the idea of bringing flowery beauty and a metaphorical smile to the cells can be uplifting.

missing image

Production: Insert Illustration 50 here.

Illustration 50. Our cells feel beautiful, like pretty flowers.

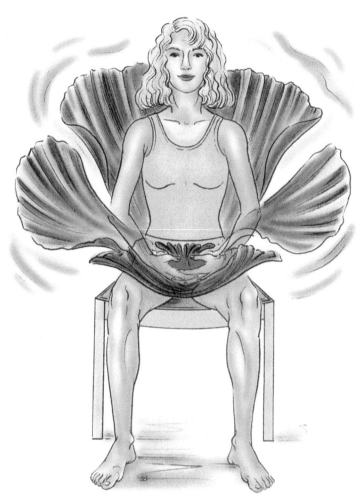

Illustration 51. Beautiful flower meditation

Peace and Serenity for Your Cells

Sometimes, simply the repetition of a single word can have a big effect on the body. For the word we are saying to have the power to actually affect something, a certain power needs to be behind the word and we have to have a physical readiness to receive the word's message. If there is neither a certain power nor a modicum of sincere willingness, one is, in the truest sense, speaking a meaningless utterance. One can test this simply by internally repeating, "tranquility and peace, tranquility and peace, tranquility and peace." Do you feel no effect or are you unsure of whether you are feeling a change (or whether it's just an illusion)? If so, it is time to assemble the power that is behind every word, and to aim to make your body and therefore your cells receptive to the words you are saying. Speaking words internally is, after all, based on evidence-based self-talk (Tod, Hardy, and Oliver, 2011). You may of course simply not like the words suggested here. In that case, you can select some of your own creation.

The first prerequisite for self-talk success is that you truly want to achieve the effect you are aiming for with your internal words. If you would rather watch YouTube than practice self-talk, the words "tranquility" and "peace" will not do the trick for you. If it is your serious intention to have more tranquility and peace in your life, the words won't fall short of their desired effect. The more peacefulness your body reflects, the more you are able to eliminate stress and the happier your body will be, and you will live longer, to boot.

Try repeating this in your mind's voice: "My words are effective; my cells are receptive to my words; my cells embody peace and vibrant health. All my cells and my entire body are fit to accomplish my plans and goals."

An Energetic Beverage for Your Cells

Rub your hands against each other for a moment and then place them on an area of your body that may feel tired or tense. If you feel great, I suggest you simply place your hands on your abdomen. Now imagine that positive energy is gushing from your hands. Imagine this energy being absorbed by your cells, as if it were just what they needed. You can compare this to drinking a delicious beverage.

In a class I was teaching, a student once said that she visualizes this image as "many small kitten tongues that are slurping milk." Obviously, this is a very personal idea, but feel free to come up with anything that gives your cells the feeling of absorbing or "lapping up" positive energy.

After the exercise, you may feel that the area of your body you touched feels stronger and more relaxed at the same time.

This is also a great exercise to apply to your face to maintain and improve your skin's youthfulness. With your touch, go to every part of your face and imagine how it absorbs energy. Do not be surprised if the regular application of this exercise shows astonishing effects.

The Cell as a Sounding Body, a Crystal, and a Light Source

Cells vibrate and pulsate, and these vibrations can be supported by music, real or imaginary. Illustration 52 depicts cells being nourished by the vibrations of a large sound-creating gong.

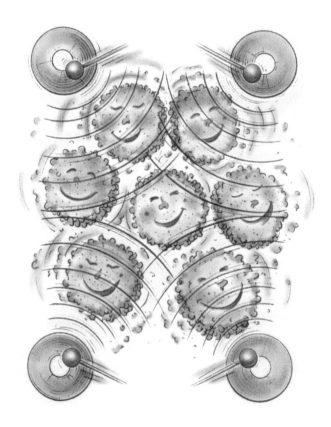

Illustration 52. Cells bathe in the vibration of a sounding gong.

As discussed earlier, cells have cytoskeletons. These cytoskeletons appear to have a crystal-like construction. Cells can modulate and break light just like crystals can. Cells can supposedly emanate very faint light in the form of biophotons and can even communicate via light (Mayburov, 2012).

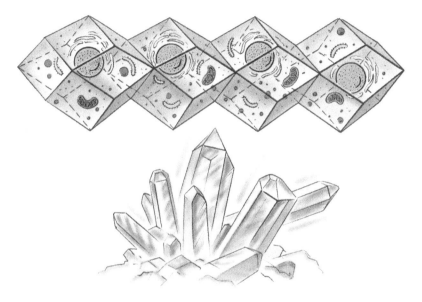

Illustration 53. Aspects of cells resemble crystalline structures, and cells can emit light.

CHAPTER 8

Youthfulness: A Question of Attitude

The conviction that all human beings get old is a very strong, irremovable, and fixated image. We see getting old as a bad thing, as something many of us fear and something that can make us sick and fragile. We are strongly convinced that the material body slowly deteriorates and then dies, because no one has proven otherwise and the evidence surrounding us is rather overwhelming; however, science states that from the cell's point of view, getting old is mainly a *program*, a *pattern*. Inside labs are living cells of people who have been dead for thirty years. There are somatic cells that can live forever in a laboratory culture, and these cells are the same as cells contained in our bodies.

Surprisingly, the aging of cells may be a relatively late invention of evolution. The first animals never died; otherwise, there would never have been evolution in the first place. Animals consist of cells, and if there are cells that don't age, then our cells have the same potential. There are, in fact, animals that don't grow old. For example, there have been jellyfish that have lived for 90 years without any symptoms of old age, until someone poured soap instead of salt into their water! There are life-forms that are far more primitive than we are that can live forever. Certain protozoa can divide themselves infinitely, for example. (Protozoa are mostly single-celled eukaryotic organisms that can move about and ingest food.)

We can also find cells that divide infinitely in our own bodies. These are the germ cells and the stem cells. Most of the body's other cells have lost this ability, however. Certain cells are programmed for aging, whereas others aren't. After approximately 50 divisions, many cells will simply die. Even if they were to be temporarily frozen for 13 years after 20 divisions, they can be reanimated but will last for only another 30 divisions, seemingly hardwired to ensure that they switch off after a specific amount of time. If one could find this "switch," one would probably live considerably longer or forever.

Whether is it desirable for humanity as a whole or for individuals to live for a long time or even forever is a philosophical debate. I will pass on that here. Our goal is to be healthy for a long time and in a natural way. Also, if we could achieve certain changes in our cellular programming without artificial medical intervention, that would certainly be a memorable achievement.

Reversing the Polarity of Our Cells

In the following mental experiment, we attempt to reverse or at least improve the programming of our cells.

First, let's establish how strongly we believe in the aging process. For this purpose, let's imagine a world in which we don't grow old, in which no one grows old, and in which health abounds for everyone. In this world, every human being can choose how old they would like to be, and when. If someone has been 20 years old long enough, that person can choose to move on to 25.

The question is, can we and do we want to imagine such a world? Do we see disadvantages? When everyone is young, one can't compare oneself to older people. Thus, where are the old and wise women and men? What would happen if I were the only one not aging? How would the people around me react when they aged but I didn't? Could I endure that? Would that be uncomfortable? Would I be afraid of envy, criticism, and suspicion? People are praised these days for looking 30 when they are 40, so society as a whole seems to appreciate such feats, but what if you would look 20 at 70? What would you choose, if you could choose?

Favorable Conditions for Living a Longer Life

Most people want to look better and feel vibrant and healthy. Improving your health and fitness takes a certain amount of effort, however, and that is where the story ends for a lot of people. Better to be unfit than to make the nutritional, mental, and physical efforts to look younger than your age would warrant.

To overcome resistance and stagnation, you need to have willpower, be self-aware, have a positive vision for yourself, and act on vision.

External behavioral patterns are often easier to change than physical and emotional patterns. Perhaps taking a look at a seemingly very healthy and fit group of people may help.

A Harvard study determined that people in Okinawa, Japan, on average live to be 81.2 years old, this being the highest average in the world. These people are very active. They hike, ride their bikes, and practice Tai Chi and karate. They also train their nervous systems by reading, drawing, and playing music, and for this purpose, they need a lot of imagination. Furthermore, they are friendly and have good relationships with their fellow people, especially with their families. They have a positive attitude toward life and can handle emotional stress well. What they don't do is just as important. They drink little or no alcohol and barely smoke, have a diet with vegetarian tendencies, and moreover don't eat much at all.

In animal testing, it has been determined that a diet reduced in calories results in the laboratory animals living longer. Overweight stresses many of the body's systems—for example, circulation and joints. Because fatty tissue is well supplied with blood, more kilograms of body weight equals more kilometers of capillary vessels through which blood needs to be pumped. One more kilogram of weight means many more kilograms of weight bearing for the knee at every step.

Nevertheless, one shouldn't associate negative imagery with any tissue in the body. At a fitness conference I recently attended, I experienced how everyone was speaking about "excessive tissue." This tissue was never labeled because it was excessive. "But there isn't any excessive tissue," I thought to myself. Every tissue we have is needed in some way; otherwise, we wouldn't have it. Certainly, the tissue mentioned in the conference was fatty tissue. Now, without a certain amount of fat, we can't live, as there are many areas inside the body where fat is indispensable—for example, on the heels as cushion, or around the kidneys as protection, and fat is an important component of the cell membrane.

To what extent fat is healthy for the body, or not, is simply a question of the amount and balance within the tissue. Incidentally, fat is said to have many stem cells, a fact that may help improve the image of the heavily discredited fat cell.

Diet is a very complex and individual matter. Every year, new approaches emerge that are supposed to help people rejuvenate and lose weight faster. In my experience, an important element on the path to success via these methods is having a positive outlook and expectation.

A Positive Image for Your Fat

We attract that of which we are afraid, because fear is associated with powerful imagery. If one is afraid of or is unsatisfied with the amount of fat on one's body, one gives the fat a lot of mental energy, and the result can be an increase in fat! Diet advertisements often have messages such as "Get rid of your fat! Never fat again!" Unfortunately, these statements may achieve the

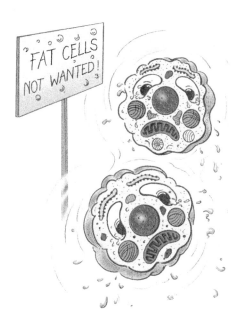

Illustration 54. Fat cells should not have a bad reputation.

opposite of the desired results, at least when it comes to mental imagery. It is impossible to imagine not-fat. What you see in your mind's eye is fat. It's probably better to think, "All my tissues are important and they fulfill their tasks diligently. I need some fat in order to be healthy." Everything is a question of balance.

Visualizing the Ideal Weight

Visualize your ideal physique and see it clearly in front of your inner eye; feel it in your body as if it were already here. Feel slender and slim, strong and flexible. Fat is our friend; we have exactly as much of it as we desire—enough to be healthy and look good. Imagine your focus on your slightly oversized belly while you're thinking you want it to vanish. This is like having a roommate you can't get rid of. Another way to look at your belly is to see it as you want it to look. Instead of putting energy into frustration, put your energy into your vision of the future.

If your diet is balanced and contains many fresh vegetables and fruit, and the usual healthy choices, and if you keep your positive vision at the forefront of your mind, you will notice that your hunger starts to adjust accordingly and your ideal weight will adjust itself as well. One reason you run to the fridge or food larder is that you have been intently visualizing what you want to eat. This is called mental training, and it psyches you up for taking action on what you are seeing. You get what you see, and if you cannot see how you want to be, then your efforts will be in vain.

Antioxidants Protect the Cells

An abundant supply of vitamin-rich foods is essential to cells' youthfulness. Instable molecules, so-called free radicals, are denounced as the cells' enemies and are besieged with antioxidants. *Antioxidant* is a general term meaning the substances that neutralize free radicals, which can harm the genetic material, the DNA, the cell membranes and other parts of the cell. Free radicals do damage by "stealing" electrons from other molecules. (Electrons are parts of the atoms that make up the molecules of which your body consists.)

Exchange of electrons is common practice among molecules, but sometimes molecules that aren't complete and are thus instable stay behind. These then become "electron thieves," known in chemistry as oxidants. Substances that provide these molecules with electrons are called antioxidants, which inhibit the oxidation of other molecules. Vitamins E and C are antioxidants, and foods such as berries, apples, onions, and greens are abundant in antioxidants.

The combination, balance, and interaction of foods is more important than excessive consumption of individual antioxidants, however. Your body produces free radicals as a byproduct of energy production in the mitochondria. In old age, the mitochondria's rate of production decreases. Their ability to convert oxygen into energy decreases, and more free radicals develop. The immune system uses free radicals as "chemical weapons" to kill off infiltrated microorganisms. In this sense, the free radicals can also be looked upon positively.

Mental Antioxidants

Let us imagine that we have just as many antioxidants in our body as we need to optimally protect our tissues. Free radicals are our friends, and they are being deployed when and where they are truly helpful. In comparison, our body always has plenty of free radicals available. Our healthy cells are untouchable and are protected by them. We always have plenty of mental vitamins E and C.

More Energy, Fewer Free Radicals

Let's imagine our mitochondria, many thousands or more in each cell. The mitochondria appreciate this attention, which gives them energy to better process oxygen and nutrients. Feel how the oxygen that we inhale is easily and entirely converted into energy.

Cell Membranes Need Fat

When the body absorbs carbohydrates or protein, these substances are broken down and put into the right shape to fit the body's needs. Several fats are broken down while others survive digestion without significant changes and become part of the cells' membranes. This fat considerably influences cellular behavior.

One of these fats is the omega-3 fatty acid. It can be found primarily in fish, certain fish oils, and some nuts and healthy seeds. Now, there's a difference between long-chain and short-chain omega-3 fatty acids, depending on the number of carbon atoms. You may have heard about the long-chain fatty acids by their abbreviations EPA, eicosapentaenoic acid, and DHA, docosahexaenoic acid. In fish, the long-chain fatty acids can be found, while most oils such as walnut, flaxseed, or hemp oils contain the short-chained fatty acids. The long-chain fatty acids eliminate inflammation-supporting molecules, and inflammatory processes make up the basis of many diseases. Different long-chain omega-3 fatty acids are also good for the heart, brain, and eyes; thus, your eating habits can directly influence the cell membrane's quality. Two issues speak against the consumption of fish, however. The first is overfishing and the resulting imminent extinction of many fish species, and the second is the high mercury content of many fish. These problems can be partly bypassed by consuming fewer big fish like tuna and focusing more on the fish in which long-chain omega-3 fatty acids are hidden, such as sardines and anchovies.

Imagining Strong Cell Membranes

Imagine strong cell membranes. Imagine them being supported by abundant omega-3 fatty acids. Imagine an abundant amount of omega-3 building blocks approaching your cells and making the membranes soft, yet strong and pliant. Imagine confident cell membranes that are excellent at performing their jobs of being flexible barriers and frontiers of communication into and out of the cells. Imagine your brain happily receiving abundant omega-3s, helping to protect itself, reconnect damaged neurons, and build stronger connectivity. Imagine your brain designating more neurons to the areas that relate to happiness, motivation, and confidence.

Exercise: Not Too Little and Not Too Much

It is well known that exercise is a very important factor for good health, yet as the ancient Greeks already knew, moderation is crucial. Too much exercise can result in stress to our bodies. I used to teach for six weeks at the American Dance Festival. Even though I generally consider dance to be healthy, in those days, I observed how something healthy could be transformed into something harmful. After about four weeks, sometimes sooner, many of the young and fit dancers had reached their limit. Many were training six hours per day with additional rehearsal hours as well. They were accordingly pale and emaciated, the result of excessive exercise. The results of too much exercise are comparable with the consequences of too little exercise: weakened immune system, reduction in strength and flexibility, and reduced confidence and stamina.

The ancient Greeks knew that balanced exercise was healthy. They essentially created the first body-mind fitness center in the world, situated in Olympia, which can still be visited today. The correlation between physical, mental, and spiritual strength was recognized and practiced. Whoever visits these sites may notice that, even today, these places appear have constructive energy and their locations are well chosen.

It is well known that exercise is beneficial for the heart and cardiovascular system. Lack of exercise is just as harmful for these organs as is smoking; however, exercise also elevates mood, improves mental performance, and possibly lowers the risk of certain cancers. Exercise helps against diabetes and should be part of the any approach to loosing weight while having a positive view of fat in your body. With sufficient exercise, muscles can better break down insulin and sugar.

If too much exercise is unhealthy, then what is the minimum? This is hard to define, but even 30 minutes of gardening per day, with good posture, of course, can count as exercise. It all depends on what you are doing. Simply contemplating the flowers, however nice they may be, will not do the trick, though walking through a natural setting at a brisk pace amidst the flowers and trees has the double benefit of being mentally uplifting and exercising.

The cells are most thankful to those who are able to perform little "exercise snacks" throughout the day. To perform these "exercise snacks," one can rely on the surrounding environment's natural conditions, such as taking exercise breaks during office hours, always walking up the stairs (knees permitting), making smaller shopping trips by bike, walking instead of taking the car, or parking your car as far away as possible from the door of the shop you are going to instead of competing for something close by. These small changes can help to create more movement in your everyday life.

Strength training is rejuvenating as well. Studies have shown that just a few months of weight training can compensate for 20 years of strength loss. Strength and flexibility also stimulate the bones and the tissue to produce new cells. You cells are simply waiting to be brought into action by your movement and your mind.

Feel Great with Movement Breaks

1.   Shoulder blades gliding on your back

The shoulder area is notorious for carrying tension, but help is on its way with the following exercise. First of all, let's think about the nature of tension. Muscle tension is a physical effort that is gripping your muscles but is not leading to any movement. Instead, it leads to feeling pained and stressed. A simply experiment can demonstrate the connection: Tense your whole body and then think, "I feel great." Obviously, there is a mismatch between your thoughts and the state of your body. Thinking that is supportive of comfort and confidence is hard to generate in a body that has tension and bad posture. You need to prepare your body to make it possible to have more useful and positive thoughts.

The shoulders need to have ample movement. When you move your shoulders, you move your shoulder blades, or scapulae. The scapula is a very popular bone, with 16 muscles or so attached to it. If the scapula is stuck on your back, the muscles will not have an opportunity to stretch and lengthen. The muscles become tense, weak, and tired, and the fascia is tight. The result is slouched posture, restricted breathing, and tight shoulders.

Lift your shoulders up and lower them back down. As you do this, imagine your shoulders sliding on your back. Metaphorically transform them into slippery bars of soap. Conjure the most lathered and soapy bar possible that slides effortlessly up and down. Move continuously and smoothly. Feel every moment and allow your breath to be effortless. You may coordinate your breathing with the movement of the shoulders, inhaling as they move up and exhaling as they drop down. If you do not like the idea of soap, imagine your shoulder blades to be surfboards gliding over waves.

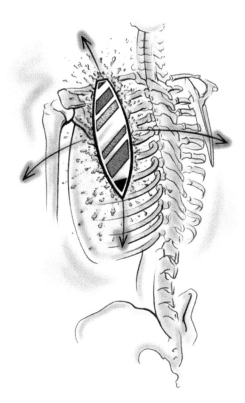

Illustration 55. Your shoulder blades are surfing.

Now shrug your shoulders to the front and to the back. This movement is also called protraction and retraction. It involves another bone, called the clavicle, which connects the scapula to the breastbone, or sternum. The clavicle is also protracting and retracting, sliding on top of your first rib. Keep breathing. Make the movement as big as possible without straining. If you have truly focused on the metaphor, you will probably have a good result as your rest and notice any changes. If you focused on discomfort, you probably will have a lesser result. Remember that much of the benefit of any exercise stems from what you are focusing on when you move.

2.   Marching on the spot

This exercise is very simple. All you do is stand and alternately lift your right and left legs. The key to this exercise is to focus on your breathing and make sure it continues smoothly and deeply throughout the exercise.

Alternately lift your right and left legs as if you were marching. Lift the knees as high as you are comfortably able to do. Do this slowly at first slowly and then accelerate. Keep going for two minutes. This does not sound like a lot, but if you really stay focused, it will nevertheless feel quite long. If you are mindlessly doing things, time flies. If you are focused, time appears to slow down. As I said, the key to this exercise is to keep breathing consciously. If you want to have another focus as well, think of smooth, lubricated hip joints. If you like metaphors, imagine strings alternately lifting the right and left knees. Keep breathing, preferably through your nose.

After at least two minutes, remain standing for several moments and observe your body. You may notice that your breath is deeper, your posture has improved, and you mind has calmed down a bit.

Healthy Vibrations

In the ancient Greek centers of healing mentioned earlier, an essential part of treatment was a beautiful environment. Flowers, plants, waterfalls, and buildings were set up in such a way that patients could take in the sights and sounds continuously. Unfortunately, most hospitals nowadays do not always embrace this philosophy. If you have ever been in a hospital, you may have found that the imagery that surrounded you may not have been the most pleasant.

We can always surround ourselves with healthy and beautiful mental energy and imagery, however. Just think of the most beautiful countryside you can mentally come up with. Absorb its relaxing and refreshing vibration. If you prefer the beach, picture that. If you like mountains, that can be the visualization you prefer. Enhance your imagery with sounds and smells. Make it come alive.

If you are good at imagery, you can also add this environment to the above exercise. In this case, you are layering activities: You are lifting your legs and focusing on your breath and lubricated hip joints while being surrounded by a beautiful environment. This is great training for your brain and body.

Bathing in the Environment We Create

We are constantly bathing in an ocean of vibrations made up of the actual environment but more primarily our own thoughts and images. This ocean contains some ice-cold currents as well as blue Caribbean waters. Before we dismiss this as nonsense, let's try this experiment.

Lift your arms up over your head and lower them again. Now repeat the movement while imagining you are surrounded by emoji-type smiley faces looking at you with happy, giggly smiles. Notice how much effort was involved in doing this.

Now surround yourself with unhappy emoji faces while lifting your arms. The emojis are scowling at you. You probably will notice a difference in the level of tension you experience in your muscles. This is a good daily practice, simply carrying your own positive environment with you. A positive environment does not have to consist of smiling emojis; it could instead be filled with beautiful flowers that surround and protect you.

The most challenging moments to your environment are when you are around negative or even angry people. This is when you can hone your practice. Keep those flowers blooming and the emojis smiling, even when adverse vibrations surround you.

Have you ever had the experience that being around certain people exhausts you, while others simply make you feel comfortable? This may have something to do with the environments they are creating for themselves, consciously or unconsciously.

Creating Our Environments

Creating our imaginary environments is much like decorating our homes, our sacred and personal spaces. Use any of the following ideas to help you decorate your imaginary home: beautiful and colorful flowers floating around you, a peaceful countryside, the sound and picture of trees rustling in the wind, crystal-clear water flowing, works of art that you like, or beautiful sounds and music filling your room. Use whatever works for you, be it floating cucumbers or butterflies.

Stem Cells: The Body's Capital

Stem cells represent the body's capital, as they can divide themselves infinitely. There are a significant number of stem cells in the bone marrow, and each produces about one to two million new cells every second. These cells convert themselves into a multiplicity of blood and immune-system cells, which are the red and white blood cells, called leukocytes, granulocytes, lymphocytes, and macrophages, and so forth.

It has been shown again and again that some patients with strong willpower can live to be cured even from life-threatening diseases. This willpower is deepened and refined by the purposeful use of thoughts and imagery. Any change in your body means a change on the cellular level. You can and are influencing your cells through your behavior, including your mental behavior.

Perhaps it is helpful to start with the statement "Anything is possible." This statement is effective because it's true: anything is possible! If you look back just 30 years, you will see that many of the things we do now may have seemed impossible then. When I started my schooling, I was writing on a mechanical typewriter. That's obviously not what I am doing now. I am of the generation that experienced the full transition to the digital world—and what a transition it was and is. And it's continuing at full throttle. Anything is possible.

Tell yourself: "In my body, anything is possible. My stem cells are happily creating new cells. Every area of my body, every tissue, is being regenerated and renewed. My cells are becoming active and dynamic in order to renew my body exactly where it is needed at the moment."

Let's speak, inwardly or outwardly, as convincingly as we are presently able to: "My genes are happy and strong; my DNA is healthy and confident. My body and all tissues are regenerating and becoming healthier from moment to moment." Then repeat as often as you feel like it: "All my tissues are becoming healthier from moment to moment."

Can Elbows Be in Love?

We often hear that the solution for tension and muscle cramps lies in more exercise; however, the secret to being relaxed, comfortable, and healthy in your body doesn't rely solely on the exercise itself but in the often-mentioned interaction of exercise, expectations, imagery, and thoughts. An exercise that effectively eliminates tension is one that is performed in an inspired way, lovingly and with joy. Love dispels tension. Love doesn't express itself only through the presence of a loved one but also in every single cell. Wherever there is love, there is no room for tension. Every movement that is performed in a unloving way may create unnecessary tension; every movement that is performed lovingly, with joy and a positive expectation, improves the fitness of your cells.

Feeling love in your body, your cells, and your muscle fibers may require a considerable amount of concentration and practice. The explanation likes in the unhappy fact that a lot of people are not happy with their bodies. Well, that is sort of like not being happy with a relationship you are in. As I mentioned above, that is a bit of a problem, because there is no way out of the relationship with your body. Separation or divorce just is not in the cards, so there is only one path forward: Appreciate the body you have and start liking it. This approach will positively change how you experience life in your body.

A lot of advertisements build on the fact that people do not like their current bodies and want to change them. This can be counterproductive, because not many people have the ideal body as depicted by magazine covers. If you are going to wait until you look like that, good luck! Start liking your body now. Say, "I like my body. In fact, it's been moving me around all my life, so thank you, body, for all that movement and for taking me places. I am looking forward to more movement in my life, with love."

I once had this experience, again at the American Dance Festival, when I accompanied some of my students to an audition for a renowned dance company. I admit to having been a bit surprised when I noticed that the dancers were not as beautiful as I had remembered them from the stage. In fact, some of them were rather short and not as lithe and long-limbed as they looked to be on stage; however, all they needed to do was dance, perform even the slightest movement, and I could see their bodies expressing love of movement. I could not take my eyes away. Those muscles and sinews were having the time of their life simply through contracting and releasing, and the joints were probably in joint heaven. Who would not like to experience joint heaven? Why do most people never get there? Probably because they do not even believe it's possible. Remember, you do not get what you want; you get what you believe. So if you want to feel great but you think you have an ugly and tight body, your imagery and your wants are not matched up.

For the sake of completion, I would like to add another story: I was once sitting next to a well-known choreographer at a dance performance, and we came to debating the performance of one of the dancers. I said, "That dancer has a great body. Why do I not enjoy watching her?" The choreographer answered, "She does have a great body, but she does not express beauty." The long-limbed and flexible body will take you only so far if the mind is not going along for the ride.

Let's take another inroad to experiencing love in our bodies and movement. Some of us have had the "butterflies," that experience of love in the belly, or of feeling love in the heart. So why not experience this also in your elbow? Why should the knee and the foot be left out of the feeling of love? Can you imagine butterflies in your elbow? I think it's a matter of simply deciding to experience love wherever we want to. Even if you have had back pain, which seems to haunt many of us now and then, why not say, "I love my back. I love my back. I love my back"? Have you ever had an argument with someone you love? Tension is really just an argument with your body's function. Deciding that we can express love, joy, and a sense of well-being in every part of the body and in every cell may be a stretch at first, even though it should be the most natural thing in the world, but not only the heart can be in love; the elbow can, too.

Send a clear message of love and joy to every tissue in your body. Your body feels your attitude toward it. If the tissue absorbs too many negative attitudes, this may, sooner or later, manifest itself in pain or, even worse, in a chronic disease such as osteoarthritis, for example. I am not questioning the mechanical factors of pain, accidents, and physical imbalances but rather am qualifying them and putting them in a larger context. We have tools at our disposal that are only a thought and an image away. Why not use them? Is it that much easier to reach for a painkiller than to use your mind and think a thought?

Love and Happiness in All My Tissues

Start by stretching and bending the fingers of one of your hands. While doing so, imagine the feeling of happiness in your tissue. Muscles, fascia, and joints are born to move; they love movement. Even your vessels and nerves participate; they have to bend and stretch a bit as well. Now move the wrist and elbow of the same arm. As you do this, say, "I love moving my body. I love moving my wrist and elbow." If a dissenting voice says,

"Baloney," ignore it. If you don't pay any attention to it, it will disappear. Keep moving.

Now add your shoulder to the action and think, "My shoulders love movement." Now move your fingers, wrist, elbow, and shoulder all at the same time. Keep going for a few moments.

Once you are done, compare the sides of your body. Which one feels more comfortable, relaxed, loving?

Now repeat the exercise on the other side.

Once you have done the other side, bring the whole body into the story and tell yourself: "I love movement. Every cell in my body loves movement." Even your breath is in love with itself; it loves movement. Your neck loves its movement. Your back and spine are thrilled to move. Your pelvis relishes every moment it can move. Your legs and feet rejoice in movement. You move your entire body and hear the cells echo the statement "We love movement!"

Smiling Cells

Imagine your cells are smiling. Smile at this moment and imagine your cells doing the same. How does this feel? What does the opposite feel like? Imagine your cells scowling.

Keeping Your Cells Flexible

Aging also relates to our cells' metabolism, such as the oxidative stress mentioned earlier. Cellular respiration consists of the cell turning biomechanical energy from nutrients into the fuel of the body, ATP. This process requires oxygen and is the reason for breathing in the first place. Cellular metabolism takes place in the mitochondria deep in the cell. To get there, the nutrients and oxygen need to travel through the cell's exterior membrane, the frontier between the interior of the cell and its environment. It is easy to imagine breathing by feeling the ribcage and abdomen move, or by sensing the movement of the lungs, but to visualize breathing at the cellular level is a different story, but this is the whole purpose of ventilating your lungs: to get oxygen to the cells to produce energy.

Let us take a moment and focus on breathing. The big question is, what does that mean? It can mean many things, and first of all, it should mean a certain kind of breathing, as in the common instruction to breathe deeply, breathe into your belly, breathe laterally, and so forth. Start your breathing experience by doing nothing but observing and sensing your breathing process. The common areas that one can sense are the movements of the belly and ribcage, but you may also feel changes in your spine, shoulders, and pelvis relating to your breathing. Now focus on the lungs, which are basically giant sponges for air. These sponges are suspended within your ribcage and are pulled outward by the movement of the diaphragm and ribs as you inhale. The lungs do not expand on their own; they are passive. Once the oxygen arrives in the lung, it travels through the very thin membranes separating the lungs from the capillaries and enters the blood.

Now move on and imagine the breathing in your cells. At this point, the oxygen is not dissolved in air but arrives carried by a red blood cell. The oxygen now diffuses through the cell membrane, which is semipermeable. You can imagine this as a sliding or slipping through the membrane rather effortlessly. The oxygen "wants" to do this, because the concentration of oxygen is lower within the cell than outside the cell. In contrast, the carbon dioxide, which is a byproduct of energy production in the cell, is higher inside the cell than outside and gets exhaled, or diffused, out of the cell into the blood. This is your cellular exhalation. Imagine the cells inhaling oxygen while they exhale carbon dioxide. At this very moment, a vast number of cells in your body are inhaling oxygen and exhaling carbon dioxide. Repeat the imagery for cellular respiration, inhaling oxygen, exhaling carbon dioxide, for at least a minute and notice how your body feels. This exercise can be very calming and may leave you with a very aerated and enriched feeling.

Fluid Cells

With increasing age, tissue becomes more and more dehydrated. That is what science tells us, but it's obviously not a great thing to imagine. If we consist of 90% water at birth, then with increasing age, up to 30% of this water is lost. Aging is drying out, one could posit.

One of the results can be the slackening of your tissues as the water-filled intercellular matrix thins out. The tissues start to "stick together." If the body's tissues, such as the layering of the fascia, start sticking together, we obviously become less flexible and our tissues sag. Remember that the matrix is the area between cells filled with collagen, elastin, glycosaminoglycans (GAGs), and fluid. GAGs are important because they attract water to become lubricants and shock absorbers for your body. GAGs help the collagen and elastin retain moisture and

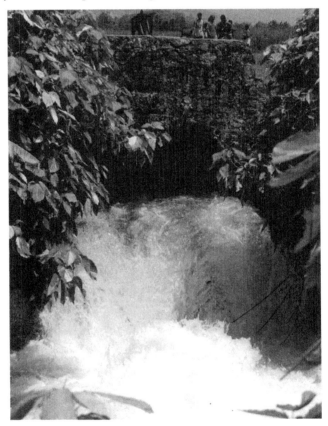

Illustration 26. Visualizing ample water in your body and matrix

increase the turgor, or bounciness, of the matrix. The matrix also forms a buffer, a sliding and connecting surface between the cells. Drinking sufficient water will help, but it's equally important to keep moving while visualizing plenty of fluid in your body. As you move, visualize your matrix replenishing itself with water. Imagine the GAGs attracting fluid, as if they were fluid sponges. Whenever you drink a glass of water, the water you are taking in increases the bounce and slide between your cells. Move any area of your body—your left arm, for example—and imagine all the cells being cushioned by the fluid matrix and sliding flexibly amongst their neighbors.

Flexible Body, Flexible Thoughts

Joints of moving surfaces are found all over the body: between the bones at the joints, between layers of muscles and their surrounding fascia, between layers of fascia, between the organs, between organs and muscles, between muscles and bones, between organs and muscles or organs and bones, between the cells, and between the cells and the matrix. The body consists of infinite sliding surfaces. If you move your arm, an infinite amount of sliding and gliding is taking place. If you move the spine, you are using an immense number of flexible surfaces. When you move your whole body, an infinite amount of sliding and gliding is taking place. Take your concept of flexibility way beyond what you ever imagined. Imagine that liquid is dancing between your cells. *Inside* the cells is liquid, *around* the cells is liquid, and *throughout* the cells is liquid. If your movement is liquid, your thoughts are liquid.

Breath Flows

Inhale and exhale deeply. Do this effortlessly as a serene observer. Imagine your breath being a wave traveling through your body. There are many ways to do this. One approach is to imagine the breath originating inside your belly and proceeding all the way up to the chest. When you exhale, this wave goes from the chest downward all the way into the belly. Observe this wave, upward and upward again, without interfering. Sometimes it is bigger, and other times, smaller. There is no good or bad, solely your breath and you as the observer.

Fragrant Oil Flexibility

Most of us have had the experience, perhaps during a massage, of rubbing oil with a nice fragrance on our bodies. Now you can combine the experience while practicing inner cellular flexibility. As you rub the oil on an area of the body, imagine that a warming layer of oil surrounds every single cell. After all, the cell membranes do consist of phospholipids. Massage any area of your body with oil, and imagine the smooth flexibility existing deep within your body and within the matrix and cells as well. Lubricate your shoulders and arms and any area that feels like it needs the experience of more flexibility.

Cellular Serenity

People who live long lives do not necessarily report easy lives but do report being able to react calmly to the ups and downs of life. An attitude that lets us enjoy life in a more stress-free manner appears to benefit longevity. Calmness isn't the same as indifference, however; sufficient calmness means not becoming agitated by every unpleasant event in life. "Things happen," we say. If we observe events while remaining sufficiently detached, it's easier for us to come up with solutions.

Now imagine calmness in your cells. Your cells feel peaceful and serene, restful and quiet. Your cells can deal with challenges in a very relaxed manner.

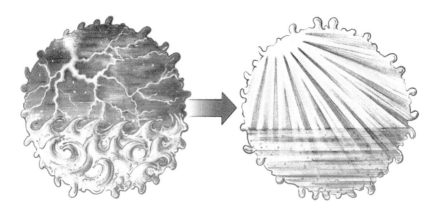

Illustration 57. Calming the storm in your cells

Calming Thoughts

Our thoughts can be seen as waves in the sea. Consciousness is like the infinite depths of the sea. A mind that is calm is like water that is undisturbed by waves. The fluid in the body is the inner ocean. Most of this fluid is located within the cells. Imagine a wavy ocean and see it become calm and quiet. Imagine the ocean within your cells going from waves to calm, restful water. Everything is at rest, and in all directions are peacefulness, vastness, and infinity.

Can We Select What's Positive?

An average day contains a lot of impressions. These inputs are recorded by the cells and by the neurons in the brain, and what the brain records becomes your heritage, but there is the possibility of being selective about the input. This selection is determined by your focus. Out of all the impressions you gather up each day, how many are positive? Do you actively seek to remember things that were positive, or do you focus mostly on a negative selection? You can start this exercise right now. Is there anything positive going on in your environment? It can be a small thing, indeed, such as an object that has a nice color or shape, or a flower.

We are not talking about glossing over problems and issues but about refraining from allowing their constant amplification to the detriment of anything positive. What impressions do you want your cells to record?

Youthful Attitude, Youthful Cells

A critical phase during aging happens when we suddenly identify ourselves with "being old" and then act accordingly. Even young people suddenly remark that they feel old. Well, yes, if you are 25, you are old compared to a 12-year-old. Notice how the statement "I am old" feels. Some people may insist and say, "But I *am* old; it's just a fact; I *am* old!" This is truly powerful mental rehearsing, only to the speaker's detriment. Many people who reach 90-plus years would take exception to this and say that they do not feel old and do not want to behave old. What about an old person behaving more like a young person—is that person out of place? I have noticed that old people who are still very resilient and sexually active are at times perceived with suspicion and even pity because they aren't acting according to their age. Is age-based behavior necessary in order to be accepted by others? Would that not accelerate aging?

Your cells can be young at any age. Simply think, "My cells are young cells. They are dynamic. They have a long life in front of them. In fact, they have the potential of immortality. That is what I choose to visualize."

One of my students was suffering from a viral heart disease. Her condition was already very serious, and doctors couldn't give her any hope of recovery. After some practice, however, she felt so comfortable in her body and her tissue that she recovered despite the incurable disease. She ascribes her healing to the great sense of well-being she had within her cells.

Your Cells Are Connected to the Entire Planet

Tremendous creative activity unfolds every moment in every corner of this planet. At this very time, countless numbers of living beings are being born, from nearly invisible jellyfish to elephants and giraffes. Trillions of flowers are unfolding themselves at this very instant, and ideas and thoughts are swirling in and around millions of human heads in the form of (hopefully) creative ideas and inspirations. During the time in which you inhale and exhale just once, the world's trees have, in total, reached 10,000 km higher into the sky. Astonishingly enough, these facts have the potential of increasing your cellular fitness if you can experience yourself as part of this orgy of creation.

We inhale what trees, plants, and endless amounts of phytoplankton in the oceans exhale. Can this give us the feeling of being fully interconnected with the planet, not related to just our families but to the whole world? The perception of your current problems may start to melt away if you can get in touch with the feeling of the energetic support that is available for your cells throughout the planet. Just imagine the enormous exchange of oxygen and carbon dioxide that is happening on the planet. Phytoplankton in the ocean and plants use carbon dioxide to creating their physical substance in a process called photosynthesis. Animals build their bodies with the help of oxygen and nutrients through respiration. Plants also use oxygen at night when no photosynthesis can take place.

As we exhale, we are nourishing plants and plankton, and as we inhale, plants and plankton are nourishing us.

Thoughts, the Energy of Our Cells

Imagine that your thoughts are the engine that runs all your cells' activity. Let us practice this by focusing on the brain.

Every second, your brain is performing thousands and thousands of complex functions. Impulses are being exchanged and transmitted with dazzling speed through a collaboration of millions of cells. Imagine that your thoughts are providing the energy that drives this activity, as if your thoughts were the wind that powers cell activity and your brain cells were millions of miniature windmills. If your thoughts are positive, motivated, and harmonious, your windmills (cells) function smoothly and efficiently and are full of positive energy.

For a few days, practice the following. Every morning for three minutes, focus on the positive influence that your thoughts are having on your brain cells. Send your brain cells some beautiful thoughts, happy imagery, relaxation, and rejuvenating ideas. Feel how this positive attitude spreads all over your body.

Nourishing Our Cells with Sunlight

Visualize a brightly glowing sun located above your head. Imagine this sun's rays penetrating and nourishing your body. The sun positively influences protein production in your cells. The sun's bright

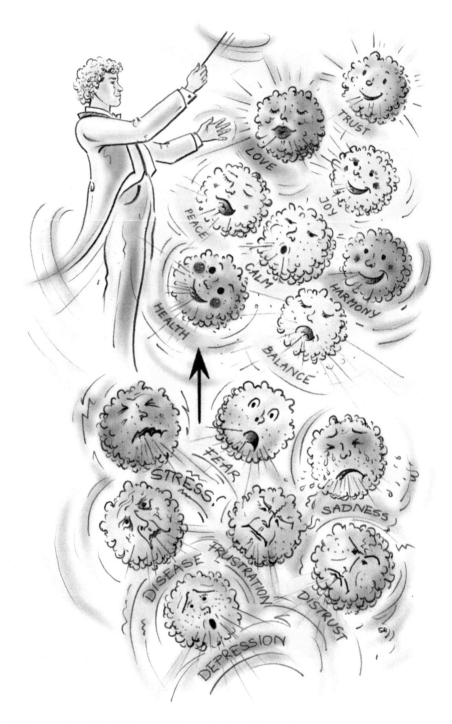

Illustration 58. The positive wind of thoughts

and warming light causes your cells to produce proteins that build and nourish your body optimally. Every tissue gets what it needs in just the right quantity.

Imagine that your DNA is in contact with the sun, being cleansed by the sun's bright, shiny light. Imagine the cells becoming brighter, reminding you of how a lantern brightens when a candle is lit inside it. This light prevents anything dark and negative from entering the cell.

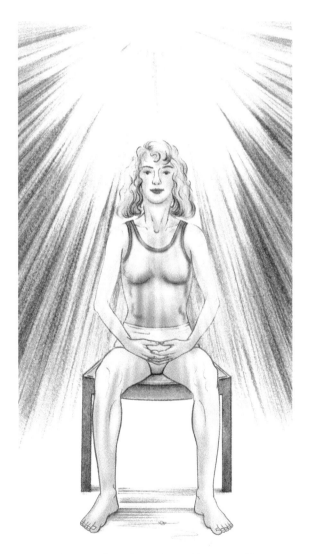

Illustration 59. The sun brightening all our cells

A Thought Massage for the Cells

Imagine that your thoughts are subtly massaging your cells. A positive, uplifting thought is an expert massage; a negative or critical thought is a painful massage. Because we are involved in our thoughts for much of the waking day, a lot of negative thinking will mean an unhappy day for your cells. Every thought can be considered a small package of vibration, a small impulse that can either help the body or even harm it. If we feel agitated toward someone else, these agitated thoughts initially affect our own tissues. Being aggravated or angry is a setback for our own tissues.

Zoned for Health

Imagine your cells to be zoned for health, an area decidedly free of any negative emotions. Weakening and disruptive vibrations are not allowed in the "healthy cell zone." If you wish, you can conjure an imaginary fence of light around each cell that keeps the cell clean and free of all negative influences. Imagine your cells communicating expertly and collaborating happily to keep you healthy and happy.

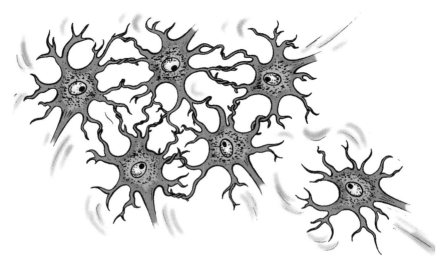

Illustration 60. Cells happily communicating and collaborating

Buckets of Thoughts

Imagine at the end of the day that you are filling up two buckets with the sum of your daily thoughts. In one of the buckets go negative or critical thoughts—anything at all aggravating. The other bucket you fill up with your happy, healthy, appreciative, grateful, and positive thoughts. Which bucket do you suppose is fuller?

I suggest doing this experiment every day for an entire week. In the evening, observe your buckets and compare them. The buckets tell us something about our mental practices. If you do not remember what kind of thoughts you had, you may want to try to do this exercise intermittently during the day; for five minutes out of every hour, notice your thoughts and decide if they are more positive and useful, or negative and detrimental. The difference is not always that clear, but in general, you will be able to make a distinction.

Can We Speak Positively About Our Bodies?

Mentally scan your body, head, neck, shoulders, arms, back, belly, pelvis, legs, knees, and feet and figure out if you have something positive you can say about each area. Can you say anything at all? Is it negative? Just imagine you're a knee and all you ever hear is that you are a pain. What if you were a disc and you heard only the worst comments and thoughts about you. Would you want to heal? "Why bother in such an unwelcoming world?" the body part may be thinking.

Have no doubt, it is important to acknowledge how you feel. If you have a painful area, you cannot just talk it away by saying there is no pain; in all but the rarest cases, that is a great misunderstanding of positive thinking. Once you have acknowledged a body area's dire state, however, it is important to move forward, have a vision, a goal, to create a positive expectation for the future. Let's give this idea a little practice.

Taking Time for Appreciation

Take a look at one of your hands and ask yourself: "What do I have say to my hand? Do I think it is brilliant, elegant, and well-proportioned? Does it work flawlessly? Does it match my arm perfectly, and does it match the rest of my body?" Imagine all the years your hand has fulfilled tasks for you, grasped things, used tools, faithfully typed and written things down, perhaps done some throwing and catching, cooking, cleaning, touching, and loving. It's an endlessly versatile part of your body, the hand. Do you take time to consciously appreciate your hand? Imagine having a friend doing all of the above for you and never thanking her. I think that person would not be your friend anymore.

Now repeat this process for the entire body. Observe your elbow and ask yourself: "What do I have to tell my elbow?" Observe your shoulders and ask yourself: "How can I appreciate my shoulders?" Observe your head and neck and ask yourself: "How can I appreciate my head, eyes, nose, and mouth?" Observe your back and ask yourself: "What do I like about my back? Anything?" Observe your abdomen and ask yourself: "What do I have to tell my belly? Only that it is not slim enough? Anything positive?" Pay attention to your pelvis and ask yourself: "What can I communicate to my pelvis for being the link between my upper and lower body and for doing all kinds of great things for me?" Focus on your legs, your knees, your feet, and ask yourself what you have to tell them. And what about the internal organs? The liver? The lung? The heart? The kidneys? And ultimately, what about your cells? Can you say anything at all that is specifically positive about your organs and cells? "Thanks!" is a beginning, but not really that exciting. Imagine doing your friend a big favor that takes a lot of time and effort and your friend says only "Thanks." Your heart beats more than one hundred thousand times a day and will likely beat more than 3 billion times in your lifetime. Is "thanks" enough for that kind of a mind-boggling achievement?

Interestingly, it is difficult for many people to express positive emotions about their bodies. If I ask a person what positive thing he or she has to share about his or her feet, the response is often a suppressed har-rumph: "They smell"; "I can't reach them"; and so forth.

It's time to resolve to appreciate our bodies and to do it more specifically. If we do this, even just a little bit, or more than we have so far, it can truly work miracles. Our cells will thank us.

References

Berk, L. S., Tan, S. A., & Berk, D. (2008). Cortisol and catecholamine stress hormone decrease is associated with the behavior of perceptual anticipation of mirthful laughter. The FASEB Journal, 22(1 Meeting Abstracts), pp. 946-11.

Bingel, U., Wanigasekera, V., Wiech, K., Ni Mhuircheartaigh, R., Lee, M. C., Ploner, M., Tracey, I. (2011). The effect of treatment expectation on drug efficacy: Imaging the analgesic benefit of the opioid remifentanil. Science Translational Medicine 3 (70, ra14), p. 70.

Dossey, L. (1995). Healing Words: The Power of Prayer and the Practice of Medicine, Harper Collins, NY.

Feltz, D. L. and Landers, D. M. (1983). The effects of mental practice on motor skill learning and performance. A meta-analysis, Journal of Sport Psychology, 5,25-57

Franklin, E. N. (2013). Dynamic Alignment Through Imagery, Second Ed. Champaign, IL: Human Kinetics.

Franklin, E. N. (2014). Dance Imagery for Technique and Performance, Second Ed. Champaign, IL: Human Kinetics.

Goldacre, B. (2013, Feb 2). Health care's trick coin. New York Times, p. A23.

Goleman, D. (1991, November 26). Doctors find comfort is a potent medicine. New York Times, Nov. 26, 1991, pp. C1, C8.

Hodges, P. W., Vleeming, A. and Fitzgerald, C. (Eds.) (2010). Strategies for motor control of the spine and changes in pain: The deep vs. superficial muscle debate; 7th Interdisciplinary World

Congress on Low Back and Pelvic Pain. Los Angeles, CA, pp. 414–419.

Hugdahl, K., Rosén, G., Ersland L, Lundervold, A., Smievoll, A. I., Barndon, R., Thomsen, T. (2001). Common pathways in mental imagery and pain perception: An fMRI study of a subject with an amputated arm. Scandinavian Journal of Psychology 42 (3): pp. 269–275.

Ingber, D. E. (1998). The architecture of life. Scientific American 278: pp. 48-57.

Ingber, D. E. (1997). Tensegrity: The architectural basis of cellular mechanotransduction. Annual Review of Physiology 59: pp. 575–599.

Kjellgren, A., Sundequist, U., Norlander, T, Archer T. (2001). Effects of flotation-REST on muscle tension pain. Pain Research and Management 6 (4): pp. 181–189.

Kross, E., Berman, M. G., Mischel, W., Smith, E. E., & Wager, T. D. (2011). Social rejection shares somatosensory representations with physical pain. Proceedings of the National Academy of Sciences, USA, 108 (15), pp. 6270–6275.

Mayburov, S. N. (2012, May). Photonic communication and information encoding in biological systems. Talk given at Quantum Information Conference, Torino.

Murphy, S., Nordin, S., and Cumming, J. (2008). Imagery in sport, exercise and dance. In T. Horn (Ed.) Advances in Sport Psychology (2nd Ed) Champaign, IL: Human Kinetics, pp. 405-440.

Panerai, A. E. and Sacerdote, P. (1997). -endorphin in the immune system: A role at last. Trends in Immunology 18 (7): pp. 317–319.

Quiroga, M. C., Bongard, S., Kreutz, G. (2009). Emotional and neuro-humoral Responses to dancing tango argentino: The effects of music and partner. Music and Medicine 1 (1): pp. 14–21.

Ranganathan, V. K., Siemionowa, V., Jing, Z. L., Sahgal, V., Yue, G. H. (2004). From mental power to muscle power—Gaining strength by using the mind. Neuropsychologia 42 pp. 944–950, 956.

Reynolds, G. (2015, July 22). How walking in nature changes the brain. New York Times.

Richardson. A (1967b) Mental Practice. A review and discussion (part 2) Research Quarterly, 38, pp. 263-273.

Ridley, M. (2003, June). What makes you who you are; Which is stronger—nature or nurture? Time magazine, p. 54

Satprem (1982). The Mind of the Cells, New York, NY: Institute for Evolutionary Research.

Syrjala, K. L., Donaldson, G. W., Davis, M. W., Kippes M. E., Carr J. E. (1995). Relaxation and imagery and cognitive-behavioral training reduce pain during cancer treatment. Pain 63 (2): pp. 189–198.

Tod, D., Hardy, J., Oliver, E. (2011). Effects of self-talk: A systematic review. Journal of Sport and Exercise Psychology 33 (5): pp. 666–687.

Recommended Reading

Alter, Michael J. (1988). The Science of Stretching. Champaign, IL: Human Kinetics.

Clark, Barbara (1963). Let's Enjoy Sitting-Standing-Walking. Port Washington, NY: Author.

Clark, Barbara (1968). How to Live in Your Axis-Your Vertical Line. New York, NY: Author.

Clark, Barbara (1975). Body Proportion Needs Depth-Front to Back. Champaign, IL: Author.

Cohen, Bonnie B. (1980–1992). Sensing, Feeling, and Action: The Experiential Anatomy of Body-Mind Centering. Northampton, MA: Contact Editions.

Dowd, Irene (1990). Taking Root to Fly. Northampton, MA: Contact Editions.

Epstein, Gerald N. (1989). Healing Visualizations. New York: Bantam Books.

Franklin, Eric N. (2013). Dynamic Alignment through Imagery, Second Ed. Champaign, IL: Human Kinetics.

Franklin, Eric N. (2014). Dance Imagery for Technique and Performance, Second Ed. Champaign, IL: Human Kinetics.

Franklin, Eric N. (2002). Relax Your Neck, Liberate Your Shoulders, The Ultimate Exercise Program for Tension Relief. Hightston, NJ: Princeton Book Company Publishers, Elysian Editions.

Franklin, Eric N. (2003). Pelvic Power: Mind Body Exercises for Strength, Flexibility, Posture and Balance for Men and Women. Hightstown, NJ: Princeton Book Company, Elysian Editions.

Hawkins, Alma M. (1991). Moving from Within. Pennington, NJ: A Capella Books

Juhan, Deane (1987). Job's Body. Barrytown, NY: Station Hill Press.

Keleman, Stanley (1985). Emotional Anatomy. Berkeley, CA: Center Press.

Kristic, Radivoj V. (1997). Human Microscopic Anatomy. Heidelberg: Springer.

Norkin, Cynthia C. and Levangie, Pamela K. (1992) Joint Structure and Function. Philadelphia: F. A. Davis.

Olsen, Andrea (1991). Body Stories: A Guide to Experiential Anatomy. Barrytown, NY: Station Hill Press.

Page, Todd and Ellenbecker S., Editors. (2003). Scientific and Clinical Application of Elastic Resistance. Champaign, IL: Human Kinetics Publishers.

Rolland, John (1984). Inside Motion: An Ideokinetic Basis for Movement Education. Urbana, IL: Rolland String Research Associates.

Sweigard, Lulu E. (1978). Human Movement Potential: Its Ideokinetic Facilitation. New York: Dodd, Mead and Company.

Todd, Mabel E. (1937). The Thinking Body. New York: Dance Horizons.

Todd, Mabel E. (1920–1934). Early Writings. Reprint. New York: Dance Horizons.

Todd, Mabel E. (1953). The Hidden You. Reprint. New York: Dance Horizons.

Index of Exercises

The Franklin Method was founded in 1994, and was originally for dancers. Extended from dance field to every kind of human movement, this method combines dynamic science-based imagery, touch, anatomical embodiment and educational skills to create lasting positive change in body and mind, using a range of simple tools, like balls, resistance bands and other daily life objects.

The Franklin Method activates body and mind function through the use of imagery, experiential anatomy and reconditioning movement to improve function.

It maximizes neuroplasticity to relearn body posture and movements by practicing movement with activation of unused musculature.

The principal goals are how to obtain dynamic body alignment and how to move the body with maximum efficiency.

In every moment, the ideal combination of limbs, joints,gravity, moving parts, connective tissue, and muscles must be found and directed by the brain and nervous system by help of appropriate imagery.

Imagery promotes a neurogenic changement of muscular condition which allows immediate results, before any myogenic (muscle tissue) one. Connective tissue and inner organs are also directly stimulated, with touch and visualization, in order to change posture and to obtain an inner and outer balance. The exercises have a considerable impact on lowering structural stress, too.

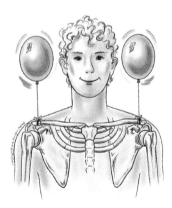

Learn more about the Franklin Method, watch free video lessons and find his other books online here:
FranklinMethod.com

And check out our online courses, to learn from Eric Franklin wherever you are:
FranklinMethodOnline.com

CPSIA information can be obtained
at www.ICGtesting.com
Printed in the USA
BVOW11s0231270417
482407BV00015B/220/P

9 781457 547065